Minimally Invasive Spine Interventions

Sang-Heon Lee
Editor

Minimally Invasive Spine Interventions

A State of the Art Guide to Techniques and Devices

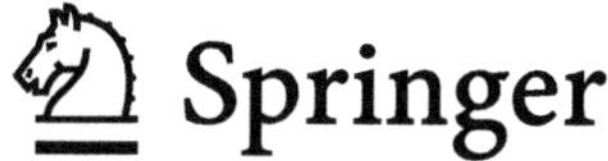

Springer

Editor
Sang-Heon Lee
Spine & Pain Center
Korea University Anam
Seoul, Korea (Republic of)

ISBN 978-981-16-9549-0 ISBN 978-981-16-9547-6 (eBook)
https://doi.org/10.1007/978-981-16-9547-6

This Springer imprint is published by the registered company Springer Nature Singapore Pte Ltd.
The registered company address is: 152 Beach Road, #21-01/04 Gateway East, Singapore 189721, Singapore

Preface

It is a great honor to present this book on interventional spine procedure.

Around the world, life expectancy in humans is rising rapidly. Elderly patients with spinal conditions suffer much less of a risk when they receive minimally invasive interventional procedures and rehabilitation compared to undertaking open surgery. It is clear which is the ideal option for treating spinal disease among the elderly.

Before the pathology causing pain and neurological deficit reaches a point where it can only be treated with surgery, it must be removed with minimally invasive methods and the patient should receive adequate rehabilitation exercise treatment. Patients are able to live the rest of their lives free of pain and disability without surgical treatments using this method.

In the past, it was very difficult to remove thickened yellow ligaments of spinal stenosis or herniated intervertebral discs that cause nerve problems. But in recent years, new medical equipment has been developed, allowing the removal of pathological tissue without significant tissue damage.

Now, both elderly patients and other patients of all ages can receive this minimally invasive treatment prior to the worsening of their conditions to the degree that surgical treatment is required.

In the future, minimally invasive spine interventional procedures and devices will continue to be developed and improved.

I have developed a medical device capable of removing herniated disc tissue itself through minimally invasive spine interventional procedure using a navigable plasma disc decompression catheter.

In order to educate others on these new minimally invasive procedures, I have conducted more than 100 lectures and live surgeries in 10 countries around the world. However, I have seen many cases where surgeons find it difficult to perform the procedure even after attending live surgery and completing cadaver practice.

I felt that a book explaining these new procedures with pictures and step-by-step instructions is absolutely necessary to help spinal interventionists perform these treatments. Physicians will find the pictures, descriptions, and step-by-step instructions found in this textbook helpful. The necessity of comprehensive instructions on these minimally invasive procedures cannot be overstated.

For this reason, I accepted without hesitation when Springer Nature proposed that I write a book on this matter.

It is my hope that through this book, spine interventionist physicians will learn the procedure more accurately, and more patients will receive the most effective treatment with minimal tissue damage instead of more invasive surgery or procedures that can cause harm to the elderly.

I deeply appreciate Dr. Richard Derby and Dr. Yung Chen who taught me spinal interventions and aided and guided me in developing a navigable plasma disc decompressor.

Finally, I would like to express my sincere gratitude to Professor Nackhwan Kim for his dedication to the completion of this book.

Seoul, Republic of Korea Sang-Heon Lee

Acknowledgments

The editors would like to thank all the contributing authors. This book was a difficult project and could not have been completed without their passion. We appreciate the time they took out of their busy clinical, teaching, and research schedules, and we are indebted to these individuals for sharing their expertise and ideal concept in the area of minimally invasive spine intervention.

We also want to thank the members of the Korean Pain Intervention Society (KORSIS) for their support and encouragement to finish the work. Their presence made it possible to start and finish this work. We wish the prosperity of KORSIS.

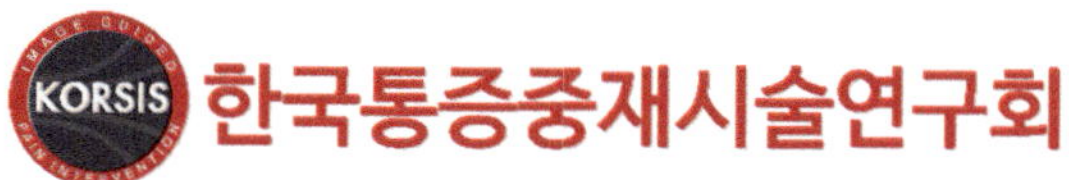

Contents

Contributors

Min Cheol Chang Department of Physical Medicine and Rehabilitation, Yeungnam University Medical Center, Daegu, Republic of Korea

Pyung Goo Cho Department of Neurosurgery, Ajou University Medical Center, Suwon-si, Republic of Korea

Yun-Woo Cho Ahn, Sang-Ho Rehabilitation Clinic, Daegu, Republic of Korea

Seong-Soo Choi Department of Anesthesiology and Pain Medicine, Asan Medical Center, Seoul, Republic of Korea

Gyu Yeul Ji Department of Neurosurgery, Yonsei Hana Hospital, Gimpo-si, Republic of Korea

Doo-Hwan Kim Department of Anesthesiology and Pain Medicine, Asan Medical Center, Seoul, Republic of Korea

Gi-Wook Kim Department of Physical Medicine and Rehabilitation, Jeonbuk National University Medical Center, Jeonju-si, Republic of Korea

Nackhwan Kim Department of Physical Medicine and Rehabilitation, Korea University Anam Hospital, Seoul, Republic of Korea

Dong Gyu Lee Department of Physical Medicine and Rehabilitation, Yeungnam University Medical Center, Daegu, Republic of Korea

Jongsun Lee Department of Neurosurgery, Nasaret International Hospital, Incheon, Republic of Korea

Jun Ho Lee Department of Anesthesiology and Pain Medicine, Jeonbuk National University Medical Center, Jeonju-si, Republic of Korea

Jung Hwan Lee Namdarun Rehabilitation Clinic, Yongin-si, Republic of Korea

Sang-Heon Lee Department of Spine and Pain Center, Korea University Anam Hospital, Seoul, Republic of Korea

Kyung-Woo Park Kwanghye Spine Hospital, Seoul, Republic of Korea

Sang Hyuk Park Yonsei Barowalk Clinic, Anyang-si, Republic of Korea

Dong Ah Shin Department of Neurosurgery, Yonsei University Severance Hospital, Seoul, Republic of Korea

Sung-Eun Sim Department of Anesthesiology and Pain Medicine, Seoul St. Mary's Hospital, Seoul, Republic of Korea

Yongjae Yoo Department of Anesthesiology and Pain Medicine, Seoul National University Hospital, Seoul, Republic of Korea

Abbreviations

ADP	Adenosine diphosphate
AF	Annulus fibrosus
AP	Anteroposterior 3
APLD	Automated percutaneous lumbar discectomy
aPTT	Activated partial thromboplastin time
ASRA	American Society of Regional Anesthesia and Pain Medicine
C	Cervical
CEI	Caudal epidural injection
CLO	Contralateral oblique
CT	Computed tomography
DRG	Dorsal root ganglion
EI	Epidural injection
ESI	Epidural steroid injection
FBSS	Failed back surgery syndrome
HIZ	High-intensity zone
HNP	Herniated nucleus pulposus
Ho:YAG	Holmium:yttrium-aluminum-garnet
IAD	Internal annular disruption
ICP	Intracranial pressure
IDET	Intradiscal electrothermal therapy
IDRA	Intradiscal radiofrequency annuloplasty
IED	Internal endplate disruption
ILEI	Interlaminar epidural injection
IM	Intramuscular
INR	International normalized ratio
IV	Intravenous
IVD	Intervertebral disc
L	Lumbar
LBP	Low back pain
LFSS	Lumbar foraminal spinal stenosis
LMWH	Low-molecular-weight heparin
MBNB	Medial branch nerve block
MPF	Motorized percutaneous foraminoplasty
MRI	Magnetic resonance imaging
N_2O	Nitrous oxide
Nd:YAG	Neodymium:yttrium-aluminum-garnet
NRS	Numerical rating scale

NSAID	Non-steroidal anti-inflammatory medication
ODI	Oswestry Disability Index
PEA	Percutaneous epidural adhesiolysis
PELAN	Percutaneous endoscopic lumbar annuloplasty and nucleoplasty
PEN	Percutaneous epidural neuroplasty
pKA	Acid dissociation constant
PLDD	Percutaneous laser disc decompression
PLF	Percutaneous lumbar foraminoplasty
PLLD	Percutaneous lumbar laser discectomy
PRP	Platelet-rich plasma
RCT	Randomized controlled trial
RFA	Radiofrequency ablation
RMDQ	Roland Morris Disability Questionnaire
S	Sacral
SAP	Superior articular process
SI	Sacroiliac
SNRB	Selective nerve root block
T	Thoracic
TELA	Transforaminal epiduroscopic laser annuloplasty
TELDA	Transforaminal epiduroscopic laser discectomy and annuloplasty
TELF	Transforaminal epiduroscopic laser foraminoplasty
TFEF	DEFINITION NEEDED
TFEI	Transforaminal epidural injection
TFESI	Transforaminal epidural steroid injection
TFL	Transforaminal ligament

Part I

General

1 Introduction

Sang-Heon Lee

A review of the history of minimally invasive spine surgery can facilitate the understanding of spinal pathology and describe the progress of its surgical treatment. Surgeons have adopted a variety of new minimally invasive technologies to improve the treatment of spinal diseases, including lasers, endoscopy, and image guidance systems. Intervertebral disc (IVD) pain is treated using chemical nucleolysis, automated percutaneous discectomy, and intradiscal thermoablation. Endoscopic procedures were among the first minimally invasive approaches to spine surgery. Spinal endoscopy is used to perform an anterior release of scoliosis, correct scoliosis deformities, and perform transthoracic microsurgical resections. Image guidance systems have been widely used for intracranial surgery, improving the accuracy of pedicle screw placement. Minimally invasive spinal surgery can be considered a small-incision approach aimed at matching the effectiveness of conventional wide-incision surgery.

Various dictionaries define the word interventional as an adjective that conveys the intent of modifying an outcome. As applied to procedures intended to diagnose or treat pain emanating from the spine or adjacent structures, the interventions are typically performed by percutaneous needle access or access requiring a minimal incision and performed using endoscopes. Needles or endoscopes are precisely guided to their target using fluoroscopy, ultrasound, CT scan, direct visualization in the case of endoscopes, or a combination thereof.

Historically and before their classification as interventional, spine surgeons typically used various endoscopic approaches to access deep spine structures. Spinal endoscopy was and continues to be used for the anterior release and correction of scoliosis deformities as well as transthoracic microsurgical resections. Over circa 40 years, the scope of practice has grown to include board-certified sub-specialists within Anesthesiology, Psychiatry, Radiology, and others. In these same years, newer interventional procedures with accompanying instrumentation, guidance techniques, and injectate solutions have evolved.

The following chapters present an overview of the precepts and techniques of interventional procedures used to treat pain emanating from the spine. The authors of individual chapters have extensive experience performing their assigned procedures, and some were instrumental in their development. Therefore, a positive bias is unavoidable as literature both pro and con could be used to justify their inclusion. Interventions such as interlaminar and transfo-

S.-H. Lee (✉)
Department of Spine and Pain Center, Korea
University Anam Hospital, Seoul, Republic of Korea

S.-H. Lee (ed.), *Minimally Invasive Spine Interventions*,
https://doi.org/10.1007/978-981-16-9547-6_1

raminal epidural injections, medial branch blocks, and medial branch neurotomies are generally accepted by most spine societies. In contrast, others such as lysis of adhesions, automated percutaneous discectomy, intradiscal thermoablation, and intradiscal injections of corticosteroids or currently available "regenerative" solutions are procedures that are evolving though promoted by various interventional societies.

2 Preparation for Minimally Invasive Spine Intervention

Dong Gyu Lee, Gi-Wook Kim, Nackhwan Kim, and Jun Ho Lee

2.1 Procedure Room Considerations

The procedure room should be spacious enough to easily accommodate the patient, entire staff, and equipment needed for the operation [1]. A sterile field and careful adherence to aseptic practices are vital elements of the procedure room [2]. The special instruments required for the procedures described in this book are detailed in the chapters covering specific procedures, and this section focuses on the basic equipment required for all interventional fluoroscopy operations (Fig. 2.1).

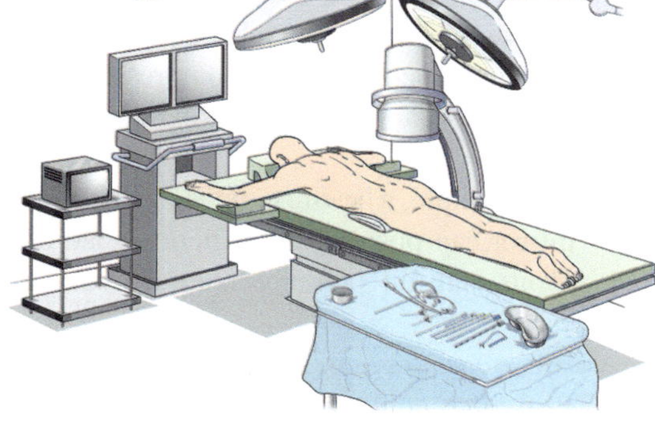

Fig. 2.1 Fluoroscopic procedure room equipment: 1, fluoroscopy (C-arm); 2, image display screen; 3, radiolucent fluoroscopic table; 4, radiation protection equipment; 5, gel or foam-made dedicated devices; 6, sterile procedure table; 7, monitoring equipment

- *Fluoroscopy (C-Arm), Image Display Screen, and Radiolucent Fluoroscopic Table* [3].
  - Fluoroscopy (C-arm): reveals the target anatomy in different projections and allows monitoring of both the needle at the target site and the contrast agent.
  - Image display screen: allows physicians to easily view the fluoroscopic images.
  - Radiolucent fluoroscopic table: allows unrestricted fluoroscope (C-arm) positioning for anteroposterior and lateral spine imaging.
- *Radiation protection equipment* [4, 5].
  - Lead aprons, leaded glass, lead gloves, mobile lead barrier shields, thyroid collars, and radiation badges.

D. G. Lee (✉)
Department of Physical Medicine and Rehabilitation, Yeungnam University Medical Center, Daegu, Republic of Korea

G.-W. Kim
Department of Physical Medicine and Rehabilitation, Jeonbuk National University Medical Center, Jeonju-si, Republic of Korea
e-mail: K26@jbnu.ac.kr

N. Kim
Department of Physical Medicine and Rehabilitation, Korea University Anam Hospital, Seoul, Republic of Korea

J. H. Lee
Department of Anesthesiology and Pain Medicine, Jeonbuk National University Medical Center, Jeonju-si, Republic of Korea
e-mail: gojuno@jbnu.ac.kr

S.-H. Lee (ed.), *Minimally Invasive Spine Interventions*,
https://doi.org/10.1007/978-981-16-9547-6_2

  - During fluoroscopic procedures, patients and physicians receive minimal radiation exposure. However, even protective lead equipment does not eliminate radiation exposure. Physicians must wear protective garments and minimize the use of fluoroscopy as much as possible to decrease their radiation exposure.
  - Radiation badges are analyzed monthly and monitor cumulative radiation exposure over time.
- *Gel or foam-made dedicated devices* [6].
  - Gel or foam-made dedicated devices provide optimal patient position for the physician to access the target area through fluoroscopic imaging and adequate space.
  - Relieve excessive local compression and improve venous return during prolonged procedures.
  - For example, a headrest made of foam with mirror can position the patient's head and avoid harmful pressure on the eyes and ears.
- *Sterile procedure table.*
  - Procedure equipment (syringes, clean linens, sterile gloves, dressing, draping, etc.) should be prepared for use within the sterile field to prevent infection.
- *Equipment for patient safety* [7].
  - Monitoring: EKG, Oximetry, Vital sign monitor.
  - Oxygen devices: Oxygen therapy, Nasal cannula, Venturi mask, Non-invasive ventilation.
  - Suction apparatus.
  - Intubation set.
  - A cart containing appropriately labeled emergency drugs (to control arrhythmias, hypersensitivity reactions, and severe hyper- or hypotension).

2.2 Intervention Documentation

Documentation serves to provide medical information about patients, including the physician's evaluation, clinical management, and procedure history [5, 8, 9]. The intervention documentation should include information obtained before, during, and after the procedure.

The pre-intervention documentation records the process of accurately determining the patient's condition and diagnosis and selecting the appropriate intervention. Pre-intervention documentation includes the patient's history (pain, medications, medical history, allergies, and contraindications to a spinal injection), physical examination (musculoskeletal and neurologic examination and diagnostic evaluation), medical decisions, and informed consent (Table 2.1). These records facilitate the selection and performance of appropriate procedures and may prevent unexpected complications.

The intra-intervention documentation records the patient's status prior to the day of the procedure and the details of the procedures. The intra-intervention documentation includes the history and physical examination, noting recent changes in the patient's status on the day, a review of systems, the anesthesia record, intervention documentation, and operative images (Table 2.2). If there is a lawsuit for an intervention-related complication, complete documentation can demonstrate that the procedure was correctly carried out [10].

The post-intervention documentation requires an overall check of the patient's condition after the intervention to ensure that the patient has fully recovered and can safely return home or to a hospital room. Additionally, a physical and neurologic examination should be performed to check for unexpected complications (Table 2.3).

Table 2.1 Pre-intervention documentation

History details about the chief complaint and present illness, the medication, medical, allergies, family, and social histories; and a review of systems should be recorded as described below		
Pain [11, 12]	Location, quality, intensity, frequency, time course, exacerbating and alleviating factors, functional status	
Medication history	Antiplatelet and anticoagulant medication use should be noted	
Medical history	Chronic illnesses	
Allergies	Previous adverse reactions to contrast require pretreatment Premedication in patients with known allergy: oral prednisolone, 20–50 mg and diphenhydramine, 25–50 mg administered 12 and 2 h before the procedure; and intravenous diphenhydramine, 25 mg provided immediately before the procedure [12]	
	Review of the patient history for any previous allergic reaction to injectants (anesthetics, corticosteroid) [13]	
Contraindications To spinal interventions	Absolute: pregnancy, infection within the procedural field, and the inability of the patient to provide informed consent [13]	
	Red flags [13, 14] (red flags should prompt an investigation of the suspected underlying pathologic condition before intervention)	Recent history of trauma Constant progressive, non-mechanical pain (no relief or worsening with bed rest) Thoracic pain History of malignancy Prolonged corticosteroid use Drug abuse, immunosuppression, human immunodeficiency virus Viral infection Unexplained weight loss Systemic illness Bowel or bladder incontinence, perianal and saddle anesthesia Fever
Physical examination [11, 13, 15]		
Musculoskeletal examination	Focused palpation or manipulation Range of motion Manual muscle test	
Neurologic examination	Motor and sensory examination (evaluating each myotome and dermatome) Neuromechanical tests (straight leg raise test, Lasegue test, Bragard's sign, contralateral straight leg raise test, femoral nerve stretch test, Valsalva test, Brudzinski test, Gaenslen test) Reflexes and pathological reflex signs Rectal and urinary sphincter function	
Diagnostic evaluation	X-ray Computed tomography Magnetic resonance imaging Myelography Bone scanning Electrodiagnostics Psychological evaluation	
Diagnosis and therapeutic intervention decisions	Physicians record the diagnosis and intervention method after a systematic patient assessment that includes the medical history, physical and neurological examinations, and various diagnostic assessments	
Informed consent	Informed consent form should be kept in the medical record after being signed by the patient in the presence of a witness [4] Elements of informed consent [16] Explain information and discussing treatment options Describe side effects, complications, and other risk factors Decision-making Signing the consent form Recording and reviewing decisions Advance care planning	

Table 2.2 Intra-intervention documentation

History taking and physical examination	Recent changes in the patient's condition, medications (especially anticoagulant discontinuation), and medical history should be reviewed before the procedure begins	
Review of systems	Vital signs including oxygen saturation, blood pressure, heart rate, and respiratory rate, and oxygen saturation should be monitored and recorded before, during, and after the procedure	
Anesthesia	If sedation is used, the patient should take nothing orally beginning 6 h before the procedure	
Intervention documentation	The patient's name and date of birth, the intervention side and site, and the planned procedure should be identified before the intervention begins [4]	
	Intervention record requirements [5, 9]	Informed consent Diagnosis Physiologic monitoring Sedation or local anesthesia Intravenous line placement (site, type) Positioning Site preparation Fluoroscopic visualization Needle placement to ensure target specificity Medications Complications Condition following the procedure
Intervention images	Fluoroscopic images obtained during the procedure should be recorded. Imaging studies in at least two planes (anteroposterior and lateral or oblique images of the fluoroscopy) should be obtained before and after the procedure. When a contrast agent is administered, post-intervention imaging should be used to record the location of the contrast material [10]	

Table 2.3 Post-intervention documentation

Checklist	Vital signs Review of systems Level of consciousness Motor and sensory function Functional status Complete anesthesia recovery
Considerations for patients with comorbidities [15]	Diabetic patients—check blood sugar levels [17] Patients with pulmonary disorders—maintain oxygen saturation above 90% Hypertensive patients—maintain systolic blood pressure below 200 mmHg and diastolic blood pressure less than 110 mmHg) Bradycardia and hypotension (close observation)

2.3 Sedation and Intravenous Lines

2.3.1 Sedation and Analgesia

Interventional procedures have been performed under sedation and analgesia recently. Sedation has the potential to render uncomfortable interventional procedures more acceptable to patients by relieving anxiety, pain, and discomfort. However, these procedures also have the risk to cause life-threatening complications, such as depression of respiratory and cardiovascular systems. Sedation has been confused with terms such as analgesia and anxiolysis. The terms are clarified in Table 2.4.

Table 2.4 Definitions [7]

Anxiolysis	Reduction of anxiety without affecting consciousness
Analgesia	Reduction of pain without mental state changes
Sedation	Controlled reduction of consciousness

Sedation is a drug-induced reduction of consciousness, a continuum ending up in general anesthesia. The American Society of Anesthesiologists defined the levels of sedation and general anesthesia and categorized four levels of sedation, minimal sedation, moderate sedation, deep sedation, and general anesthesia (Table 2.5).

Since sedation is a continuous phenomenon, it may be impossible to predict how the patient will react. Therefore, physicians should be pre-

Table 2.5 Depth of drug-induced sedation, analgesia, and general anesthesia [18]

	Minimal sedation (anxiolysis)	Moderate sedation (conscious sedation)	Deep sedation	General anesthesia
Responsiveness	Normal response to verbal commands	Purposeful[a] response to verbal or tactile stimulation	Purposeful[a] response after repeated or painful stimulation	Unarousable, even with painful stimulus
Airway	Unaffected	No intervention required	Intervention may be required	Intervention required
Spontaneous ventilation	Unaffected	Adequate	May be inadequate	Inadequate
Cardiovascular function	Unaffected	Usually maintained	Usually maintained	Impaired

[a]Reflex withdrawal from a painful stimulus is not considered a pain response

pared to resuscitate patients whose level of sedation becomes deeper than intended [19]. Conscious sedation is considered a safe target state because ventilation is within normal range, and cardiovascular function is stable. However, if verbal responsiveness is lost and the patient becomes deeply sedated, then ventilation may become inadequate. Deep sedation requires the same level of support as general anesthesia.

Intravenous (IV) sedative and analgesic drugs should be administered at an appropriate incremental doses that adjusts to the desired analgesia and sedation goals, and the administering clinician should be familiar with patient characteristics that could alter the response to treatment [18]. Sedation-related features of the medical history include the following:

1. Major organ system abnormalities.
2. Previous adverse response to sedation, analgesia, and regional and general anesthesia.
3. Drug allergies, current medications, and potential drug interactions.
4. Time and nature of the last oral intake (Table 2.6).
5. History of cigarette, alcohol, or drug use or abuse.

Patient monitoring is important in sedated patients. Monitoring improves the clinical efficacy of sedation and analgesia and reduces adverse outcomes after sedation. The recommended intraoperative monitoring after sedation is described in Table 2.7. Monitoring should continue until the patient can respond consciously to all verbal commands.

Patients should be evaluated for suitability for discharge from the clinics after sedation, because remaining sedation and cardiopulmonary depression during the recovery phase may occur. Recovery room requirements include the following [18]:

Table 2.6 Fasting recommendation to reduce the potentials of pulmonary aspiration[a] [20]

Ingested material	Minimum fasting period (hours)
Clear liquid	2
Breast milk	4
Infant formula	6
Non-human milk	6
Light meal	6

[a]These recommendations apply to healthy patients who are undergoing elective procedures and do not guarantee complete gastric emptying

Table 2.7 Recommended intraoperative monitoring after sedation [18]

1. Level of consciousness	Monitoring of patient response[a] to verbal command or tactile stimulation
2. Breathing	Observation and auscultation
3. Pulse oximetry	With appropriate alarms
4. Blood pressure and heart rate	Measured every 5 min
5. Electrocardiogram	Necessary when dysrhythmias are anticipated
6. Capnography	Monitor exhaled carbon dioxide during moderate and deep sedation

[a]The withdrawal action from a painful stimulus is not considered a relevant response

1. Medical observation of recovery and discharge.
2. A recovery area equipped with appropriate monitoring and resuscitation equipment.
3. The level of monitoring should be individualized, and monitoring should continue until appropriate discharge criteria are met.
4. Level of consciousness, vital signs, and saturation should be recorded at regular intervals.
5. Recovery room personnel should be trained to treat known complications.

If the patient will be discharged from the hospital after sedation or analgesia, the following discharge criteria should be met [18]:

1. The patient should be alert and oriented.
2. The patient's vital signs should be stable.
3. Discharge fitness scoring systems should be used.
4. Sufficient time (up to 2 h) should elapse after the last administration of reversal agents (naloxone, flumazenil).
5. Outpatients should be discharged with a responsible accompanying guardian.
6. Physicians should provide written instructions regarding diet, medications, and activities and an emergency phone number to outpatients.

2.3.2 Drugs Used for Sedation

When selecting sedatives and analgesics, and risks and benefits should be considered based on the patient's general condition. The ideal drugs can provide adequate analgesia, anxiolysis, amnesia, and somnolence. The effects, side effects, and advantages of the most frequently used medications are described in Tables 2.8 and 2.9 [7, 21].

In general, IV injection is the most commonly selected method of administration for sedation because it is the fastest and most reliable. However, if IV access is difficult, intramuscular injection or oral administration is also possible. IV injection is very effective in a very short time, but even a small dose may cause complications such as respiratory depression depending on the situation.

Fentanyl is the most commonly used opioid for sedation and analgesia. The advantages of fentanyl are that the onset is fast, the duration is long, and it does not release histamine. Respiratory depression and hypotension may occur in elderly patients or patients in poor condition. The effect of fentanyl can be reversed with naloxone. Morphine is less frequently used because of its delayed onset and short duration of action and released histamine. However, it has a

Table 2.8 Sedatives and analgesics frequently used for minimally invasive procedures

Medication	Categorization	Main effect	Administration route	Dose
Fentanyl	Opioid	Analgesia	IV	0.5–1.5 mcg/kg
Morphine	Opioid	Analgesia	IV IM	0.03–0.15 mg/kg 0.05–0.2 mg/kg
Midazolam	Benzodiazepine	Sedation/amnesia	IV IM	0.01–0.1 mg/kg 0.07–0.15 mg/kg
Ketamine	Phencyclidine derivative	Sedation/amnesia / analgesia	IV IM	1–2 mg/kg 3–5 mg/kg
Etomidate	Imidazole derivative	Sedation/amnesia	IV	0.2–0.5 mg/kg
Propofol	Alkyl phenol derivative	Sedation/amnesia	IV	0.5–1 mg/kg 2.5–15 mcg/kg/min
Nitrous oxide	Medical gas	Analgesia	Inhalation	30–60%
Dexmedetomidine	α_2-agonist	Sedation/analgesia	IV	1 mcg/kg (initial) 0.2–0.7 mcg/kg/h

IV intravenous, *IM* intramuscular

Table 2.9 Benefits and side effects of frequently used sedatives and analgesics

Drug	Administration method	Onset of action (min)	Duration (min)	Advantages	Complications
Fentanyl	IV IM	1–2 10–30	30–40 60–120	Rapid onset Short duration Rare histamine release Minimal cardiovascular effects Reversed by naloxone	Respiratory depression
Morphine	IV	10	240–360	Long-acting	Respiratory depression Hypotension Low fat solubility Slow onset
Midazolam	IV IM	1–2 10–15	30–60 60–120	Fast-acting Short duration Easy titration	Respiratory depression
Ketamine	IV IM	1 5	15 15–30	Preserved airway reflex No respiratory depression	Emesis Laryngospasm Increased ICP
Etomidate	IV	1	5–10	Rapid onset Short duration Minimal cardiovascular effects	Respiratory depression Myoclonus Adrenal suppression
Propofol	IV	<1	8–10	Rapid onset Short duration Antiemetic	Respiratory depression Hypotension Injection pain
Nitrous oxide	Inhalation	1–2	3–5	Rapid onset Short duration Minimal cardiovascular effects	Air expansion in closed body cavity Emesis
Dexmedetomidine	IV	10	120–150	Sedative + analgesic Sympatholytic Minimal cardiovascular effects	Hypertension (initial) Hypotension and bradycardia (late)

min minutes, *IV* intravenous, *IM* intramuscular, *ICP* intracranial pressure

cumulative effect and may be suitable for chronic pain control in cancer patients.

Benzodiazepines have good hypnotic and anxiolytic effects. However, they have no analgesic effect, so it can be used with opioids. Midazolam is the most frequently used benzodiazepine because its onset is rapid and duration is relatively moderate. In elderly patients or alcoholic patients, the effect of the drug may enlarge even at small doses.

Ketamine has distinct effect that induces dissociative anesthesia. There is no respiratory depression, and airway reflex is preserved. Blood pressure is not decreased. Hallucination and psychiatric problem may occur. Etomidate is a sedative agent with short duration, and has no analgesic effect. There is no effect on the cardiovascular system, so blood pressure does not drop. Respiratory depression, myoclonus, nausea, and vomiting may occur.

Propofol is the most frequently used hypnotic sedative drug. It has rapid onset, short duration, and antiemetic effect. When propofol is used with opioid, respiratory depression and hypotension may occur. There are complaints of very severe pain during injection.

Nitrous oxide (N_2O) is an inhaled agent, but it is rarely used in sedation and analgesia for minimal invasive procedure. It is acceptable analgesic in conjunction with supplying oxygen, and the

Table 2.10 Antagonists for opioid and benzodiazepines

Drug	Antagonizes	Time to effect (min)	Duration (min)	Administration method	Dose (mg)
Naloxone	Opioids	Fast	15–30	IV	0.1–0.2 (up to 1–2)
Flumazenil	Benzodiazepine	1–2	45–90	IV	0.1–0.2 (up to 1)

min minutes, *IV* intravenous

concentration of N_2O is 30–70% with oxygen. It has a good analgesic effect, but hypoxemia may occur.

Dexmedetomidine is an α_2-adrenergic agonist and has sedative, anxiety-reducing and analgesic effects. It has short duration and is mostly administered through IV infusion. Hypertension may occur in the initial phase of injection, but hypotension and bradycardia may occur later.

Sedative drugs should be carefully titrated, but the effect can last longer in some patients. In that case opioids and midazolam can be antagonized by naloxone and flumazenil.

Naloxone antagonizes respiratory depression following opioid use. Since the drug effect lasts 15–30 min, observation should be required more than 30 min after injection. Flumazenil is an antagonist of benzodiazepine. It is used when respiratory depression occurs after midazolam injection. If the effects of benzodiazepine persist, re-sedation is likely to occur when the flumazenil effect is over. The time to effect, duration, and dose of the most frequently used antidotes for agents used in sedative analgesia are described in Tables 2.10.

2.3.3 Intravenous Access

IV access is not typically required for minimally invasive procedures unless sedation is required. The IV administration of sedatives increases patient satisfaction with sedation and decreases the incidence of adverse outcomes.

Intravenous line should be secured throughout the procedure in patients receiving IV sedatives and analgesics. If the IV line becomes occluded, access should be reestablished. It is advisable that securing IV line until patients maintains stable breathing, because it allows to cope with the adverse outcome after sedation [18].

2.4 Precautions in Patients with Comorbidities

2.4.1 Scope

The indications for spinal pain management interventions are expanding, and the number of patients undergoing these procedures is increasing because of population aging. Additionally, diabetes, cardiovascular diseases such as hypertension and heart failure, and degenerative musculoskeletal disorders have a high morbidity rate.

2.4.2 Epidural Steroid Injection in Patients with Diabetes Mellitus

Reports indicate that hyperglycemia is a side effect of an epidural steroid injection (ESI) [17]. Many studies have demonstrated that the effects of corticosteroids are opposite to those of insulin, and corticosteroids increase gluconeogenesis in the liver and reduce glucose absorption in peripheral tissues [22]. Insulin sensitivity has been reported after an ESI, and one study found that glucose tolerance was altered in 10 healthy nondiabetic patients who received a caudal ESI (triamcinolone, 80 mg). Glucose and insulin levels increase significantly 24 h after a steroid injection and return to normal 1 week later [23]. One study found that epidural administration of 15 mg of dexamethasone acetate induced a systemic effect, and a single injection resulted in transient adrenal suppression, indicating that corticosteroids pass into the bloodstream [24]. Another study found a statistically significant increase in blood glucose that peaked at 106 mg/dL at baseline the evening after the injection and lasted 2 days in diabetic patients who received lumbar epidural betamethasone injections [17].

The therapeutic value of corticosteroid treatment is accompanied by known complications. The most commonly reported corticosteroid-induced side effects are rash, fever, insomnia, hot flashes, headache, and nausea [25]. Additionally, glucocorticoids act as insulin antagonists and inhibit peripheral glucose intake while promoting hepatic gluconeogenesis [26]. For this reason, clinicians must carefully monitor blood glucose levels for at least 2 days after an ESI is performed in a patient with diabetes and modify the diet and drug administration as needed. Further, physicians should consider the use of low-dose corticosteroids when performing ESIs in patients with diabetes.

2.4.3 Spinal Pain Management Intervention in Patients with Cardiovascular Disorders

Spinal pain management interventions may increase the risk of clinically significant hypotension, which can increase the risk of death or a major cardiovascular event in patients with cardiovascular disease. However, using randomized trials to investigate the effects of nerve blocks has proved difficult.

A review of cardiovascular physiology and spinal cord anatomy can reveal the mechanism of intervention-related hypotension and bradycardia. These physiological deviations are symptoms of anesthetized spinal sympathetic nerve fibers. Importantly, as the nerve block expands to higher thoracic spinal cord levels, the ability to compensate for physiological perturbations is gradually attenuated. As the T1 to L1 spinal nerve fibers are blocked, nerve signals to the adrenal gland are weakened, interfering the normal catecholamine response to low blood pressure and slow cardiac output. Sensory blocks above T4 eliminate compensatory vasoconstriction of upper extremities, and those involving T1 to T5 sympathetic fibers limit reflex tachycardia and reduce myocardial contractility. Compensatory mechanisms can be further compromised by autonomic disturbances, as found in patients with diabetes mellitus and old age [27].

The typical T4 sensory block significantly reduces the mean arterial pressure (−33% ± 15%) due to a 26 % decrease in systemic vascular resistance and a 10 % decrease in cardiac output. Nonetheless, assuming that adequate vascular pressure, contractile support, or both are provided, the effect on overall cardiac performance is minimized [28].

Spine-origin bradycardia is the result of the parasympathetic dysfunction, which occurs, in part, secondary to the blockade of cardiac sympathetic fibers from T1 to T5 but mainly due to decreased preload. Decreased intracardiac volume, pacemaker receptor responses, and left ventricular volume are thought to cause severe bradycardia and low systolic pressure through paradoxical activation of the Bezold-Jarisch reflex [27].

In one post-mortem study, a neuraxial block in patients with a high risk of postoperative cardiovascular morbidity was associated with combined primary outcomes (cardiovascular death, non-fatal myocardial infarction, and non-fatal cardiac arrest) and an increased risk of myocardial infarction, but not stroke, non-cardiovascular death, or clinically significant hypotension [29]. Importantly, conscious patients can promptly alert the physician of compromised organ perfusion by complaining of nausea or dizziness.

In another systematic review, the probabilities of pneumonia and myocardial infarction were significantly reduced in patients undergoing epidural pain therapy compared to without the therapy. However, serious adverse effects of epidural analgesia have been reported, including the risk of hypotension [30].

Bradycardia and hypotension are relatively common complications of epidural injection therapy but are not always clinically important. Cases of bradycardia not associated with hypotension that show gradual heart rate stabilization to within 10–15% of the baseline should be closely monitored but may not require treatment. However, in patients with hypertension, coronary artery disease, or underlying aortic stenosis, prompt action is required if hemodynamic abnormalities occur after the procedure [31].

Hypotension and bradycardia are common sequelae of spinal epidural intervention, and they have a propensity to cause sudden and unpredictable major hemodynamic compromise. In cases of hemodynamic compromise, the treatment goal is reversing the physiological perturbations leading to cardiac output disorders, such as decreased systemic vascular resistance, reduced preload, decreased heart rate, and decreased myocardial contraction. A substantial sensory nerve blockade, old age, and preoperative beta-adrenergic blockers are risk factors for spinal hypotension and bradycardia. However, these complications are not entirely predictable, based on the presence or absence of these risk factors. Prophylactic volume loading and vascular compression of lower extremities alone are insufficient to prevent these complications of spinal procedures. Ultimately, accurate continuous patient monitoring and comprehensive resuscitation equipment can minimize sequelae and normalize organ function.

2.5 Anticoagulants

2.5.1 Introduction

Pain-related procedure guidelines are essential because the procedural and anatomical considerations for pain intervention are significantly different from peripheral local anesthesia techniques. The goals of interventional spine and pain procedures are much wider than those of local anesthesia. Pain-related procedures range from minimally invasive procedures in high-risk subjects to low-risk peripheral nerve blocks. The American Society of Regional Anesthesia and Pain Medicine (ASRA) regional anesthesia and guidelines for acute pain are divided into three categories according to the risk of bleeding during the intervention [32] (Table 2.11).

Table 2.11 Pain procedure classification according to the potential risk of serious bleeding

High-risk	Spinal cord stimulation Dorsal root ganglion stimulation Intrathecal catheter and pump Vertebroplasty and kyphoplasty) Percutaneous decompressive laminotomy Epiduroscopy and epidural decompression
Intermediate-risk[a]	Interlaminar ESIs (cervical, thoracic, lumbosacral) Transforaminal ESIs (cervical, thoracic, lumbosacral) Cervical[b] facet MBNB and RFA Intradiscal procedures (cervcial, thoracic, lumbar) Sympathetic blocks (stellate, thoracic, splanchnic, celiac, lumbar, hypogastric) Trigeminal and sphenopalatine ganglia blocks
Low-risk[a]	Peripheral nerve blocks Peripheral joint and musculoskeletal injections Trigger point injections including piriformis injection Sacroiliac joint injection and sacral lateral branch blocks Thoracic and lumbar facet MBNB and RFA Peripheral nerve stimulation trial and implant[c] Pocket revision and implantable pulse generator/intrathecal pump replacement

ESI epidural steroid injection, *C* cervical, *T* thoracic, *L* lumbar, *S* sacral, *MBNB* medial branch nerve block, *RFA* radiofrequency ablation

[a]Patients with a high risk undergoing low- or intermediate-risk procedures should be treated as intermediate or high risk, respectively

[b]There is abundant neck vascularity in the adjacent region of the target structure

[c]Peripheral neuromodulation has a risk depending on the location of the target nerve to important vessels and the invasive intensity of the procedure

2.5.2 Aspirin and Non-steroidal Anti-inflammatory Drugs

The ASRA and European guidelines recommend performing neural blocks in patients using aspirin or non-steroidal anti-inflammatory medications (NSAIDs) [33, 34]. The Nordic guidelines for neuraxial blocks in individuals taking aspirin provide recommendations based on the reason for aspirin utilization and the daily dosage [35]. For individuals taking aspirin for secondary prevention of recurrence, the recommendation is to stop this medication up to 12 h before a neuraxial block is performed. For individuals taking aspirin for reasons other than secondary prophylaxis, the cessation period is 3 days unless the dose exceeds 1 g per day, in which case the period of rest can be extended to 1 week. For NSAIDs, the Nordic guideline recommendations are based on the specific half-life of each drug.

NSAIDs are used for symptomatic control and, unlike aspirin, do not provide heart and brain protection. Therefore, these medications can be discontinued without negatively affecting the cardiac and brain functions. Further, NSAID cessation may be required before high-risk interventional pain procedures in patients with high bleeding risk. Recommendations are based on the pharmacokinetics and associated half-life of each drug (Table 2.12). A period of five half-lives is sufficient to stop the NSAID effect on platelets. It is not necessary to discontinue cyclooxygenase-2-selective inhibitors because they do not affect platelet function.

Aspirin discontinuation is recommended before high-risk procedures with an increased risk of bleeding and sequelae in patients using aspirin for primary prophylaxis. Additionally, aspirin discontinuation should be considered before certain intermediate-risk procedures with an increased risk of bleeding, including interlaminar cervical ESIs and stellate ganglion blocks. In cases where aspirin is administered for secondary prevention, risk management decisions should be based on the shared assessments of the interventionist, patient, and prescribing physician and fully documented. The risk of bleeding with continued aspirin administration should be compared with the cardiovascular risk of aspirin cessation. In cases where aspirin is discontinued, the time of medication interruption should be determined individually. In patients taking aspirin for secondary prevention, aspirin should be stopped at least 6 days before a procedure that may present a high risk of bleeding or serious sequelae. In low- or intermediate-risk procedures involving aspirin discontinuation, this period can be shortened to 4 days to balance the benefit of bleeding prevention with the risk of cardiovascular events. In most patients, platelet function is restored 4 days after aspirin discontinuation [36].

Following a high-risk procedure, aspirin can be restarted 24 h later, if necessary, for secondary prevention of recurrence of prior cardiovascular accident, and NSAIDs should be withheld for 24 h as they are not essential for cardiovascular protection. In patients receiving aspirin for primary prevention, it should not be restarted for at least 24 h after high-risk procedures and certain intermediate-risk procedures, including interlaminar cervical ESIs and stellate ganglion block, which increase the risk of bleeding. This delay is recommended because aspirin administration affects platelet function rapidly and significantly.

Table 2.12 Chemical half-lives of commonly administered non-steroidal anti-inflammatory drugs

Agent	Half-life (hours)	Recommended discontinuation time (days)
Diclofenac	1–2	1
Etodolac	6–8	2
Ibuprofen	2–4	1
Indomethacin	5–10	2
Ketorolac	5–6	1
Meloxicam	15–20	4
Nabumetone	22–30	6
Naproxen	12–17	4
Oxaprozin	40–60	10
Piroxicam	45–50	10

2.5.3 Adenosine Diphosphate Receptor Inhibitors

Adenosine diphosphate (ADP) receptor inhibitors are used to treat coronary syndromes, cerebral vascular ischemic events, and peripheral vascular diseases. They are used in combination with aspirin, in the so-called dual antiplatelet therapy, to reduce thrombosis in patients with acute coronary syndrome after a percutaneous coronary intervention [37]. The ASRA and European guidelines recommend a 7-day interval between clopidogrel cessation and a procedure, while the Nordic directive indicates that 5 days is appropriate. The Nordic guideline is based on a 10–15% ratio of new platelets daily and a 50–75% ratio of platelets with normal function 5 days after antiplatelet drug discontinuation [38]. The Nordic guidelines recommend post-procedure antiplatelet resumption after catheter removal, while the European guidelines recommend resuming antiplatelet drugs 6 h after catheter removal. Clopidogrel can be restarted 12–24 h after spinal surgery. The ASRA guidelines recommend a 24-h interval before resuming prasugrel or ticagrelor, considering their fast-antiplatelet effects.

The ASRA guidelines suggest that low-risk procedures can be safely performed without stopping ADP receptor inhibitors, while clopidogrel should be stopped 7 days before intermediate- and high-risk procedures. Risk factors of thromboembolism include the simultaneous use of multiple antiplatelet drugs, old age, progressive liver or kidney disease, and a history of abnormal bleeding. In patients at a high risk for thromboembolism, a 5-day interval between clopidogrel cessation and the procedure is recommended, and a platelet function test should be performed if possible. Following the discontinuation of clopidogrel, prasugrel, or ticagrelor, "bridge" therapy with low-molecular-weight heparin (LMWH) may be administered to patients with a high thromboembolism risk. LMWH should be discontinued 24 h before the interventional procedure.

2.5.4 Oral Warfarin

The option to stop warfarin should be considered with the prescribing physician before low-risk procedures. Several guidelines suggest that these procedures are safe when there is a therapeutic international normalized ratio (INR) (INR < 3.0) [39]. Warfarin should be discontinued for 5 days, and the normalization of INR (≤1.2) should be confirmed before high-risk and intermediate-risk procedures. Warfarin can be restarted the day after the procedure.

2.5.5 Intravenous Heparin

Unfractionated heparin inactivates factors IIa, Xa, and IXa. The half-life of heparin is 1.5 to 2 h, and the therapeutic effect takes 4 to 6 h after administration. Heparin effects are monitored using the activated partial thromboplastin time (aPTT), and therapeutic anticoagulation is achieved when the aPTT is 1.5 to 2.5 times the initial value.

IV heparin should be discontinued for at least 6 h before performing low-, intermediate-, or high-risk pain management procedures and should not be resumed for at least 2 h after the intervention. Following an intermediate- or high-risk procedure, especially one with substantial blood loss, heparin should not be resumed for 24 h.

2.5.6 Subcutaneous Heparin

The anticoagulant effect of low-dose heparin with subcutaneous route of 5000 units every 8–12 h is caused by inhibition of heparin mediation of activated factor Xa. Maximal anticoagulation is observed within 40–50 min after administration of heparin, and the effect wears off within 4–6 h. A 6-h interval between the administration of subcutaneous heparin and an intermediate-risk intervention is necessary, while a 24-h interval and aPTT normalization are recommended before high-risk procedures. Subcutaneous heparin can be resumed at least 2 h after low-risk procedures and 6–8 h after intermediate- and high-risk procedures.

2.5.7 Low-Molecular-Weight Heparin

The plasma half-life of LMWH ranges from 2 to 4 h after IV injection and 3–6 h after subcutaneous injection. The ASRA guidelines recommend a 12-h interval between the discontinuation of prophylactic enoxaparin and a low-, intermediate-, or high-risk interventions. When using a

Table 2.13 Discontinuation and resumption of the new anticoagulants

	Half-life (hours)	Recommended interval between drug discontinuation and pain procedure (5 half-lives)[a] (days)	Recommended interval between procedure and drug resumption[b] (hours)
Dabigatran	12–17	4	24
Rivaroxaban	9–13	3	24
Apixaban	15.2 ± 8.5	3	24
Edoxaban	9–14	3	24

[a]Given the added risks in patients with chronic pain (elderly, spinal stenosis) and the surgical characteristics of some pain interventions, we recommend an interval of five half-lives between the last administration of drug and intermediate- and high-risk interventions

[b]Procedures include intermediate- and high-risk interventional pain management procedures Shared decision-making should be utilized for low-risk procedures; a 2-half-life interval may be considered

therapeutic dose of enoxaparin (1 mg per kg), the guidelines recommend a 24-h interval between discontinuation and the interventions. LMWH may be resumed 4 h after low-risk interventions and at least 12 h after intermediate- and high-risk interventions. Medications that affect hemostasis (antiplatelets, NSAIDs, selective serotonin reuptake inhibitors, other anticoagulants) should be used with care in patients receiving LMWH.

2.5.8 New Anticoagulants: Dabigatran, Rivaroxaban, Apixaban, and Edoxaban

New anticoagulants have a short half-life and do not require continuous coagulation monitoring. The ASRA guidelines recommended a two to five half-life interval between drug discontinuations and a procedure (Table 2.13).

2.6 Injectates

2.6.1 Local Anesthetics

Local anesthetics are widely used and generally safe for spine interventions and can be used for both diagnostic and therapeutic purposes. A local anesthetic injection is typically the preliminary step before nerve ablation. Immediate pain relief after the administration of local anesthetics is diagnostic information that limits the differential diagnosis by identifying the pain generator. Local anesthetics are frequently used in combination with steroids in spine interventions such as ESI. However, the therapeutic effect of these procedures is the result of the local anesthetic [40, 41].

Amide local anesthetics very rarely cause an allergic reaction, so they are widely used for spinal injections [42]. Methylparaben is a preservative that can act as an allergen; thus, preservative-free local anesthetics are recommended for epidural injections (EIs) [43]. Amide local anesthetics are hydrolyzed to inactive products by hepatic microsomal enzymes.

2.6.1.1 Mechanism of Action

Local anesthetics are weak bases with ionized (positive charge) and non-ionized forms. The non-ionized form is lipid-soluble and able to penetrate the nerve sheath. Therefore, the higher the concentration of the non-ionized form of a local anesthetic, the faster it will take effect. Each local anesthetic has a unique acid dissociation constant (pKa) pH at which there are equal amounts of the ionized and non-ionized forms. Compared to local anesthetics with a higher pKa, those with a pKa close to physiologic pH have a higher concentration of non-ionized molecules and take effect more quickly [44]. For example, the pKas of lidocaine and ropivacaine are 7.8 and 8.1, respectively, and lidocaine acts faster than ropivacaine. Sodium bicarbonate increases the pH, which increases the concentration of non-ionized local anesthetic and decreases the time to anesthesia onset, thereby improving the quality of the block [45]. The non-ionized form of a local anesthetic penetrates the plasma membrane, converts to the ionized form, and blocks the activated sodium channel inside the cell [46]. Inactivated sodium channels prevent the initiation or propagation of nerve fiber electrical impulses.

Local anesthetics undergo metabolism by hepatic microsomal enzymes. Therefore, the rate of clearance of local anesthetics from plasma is directly related to hepatic blood flow. Congestive heart failure and hepatic disease can decrease the metabolism of local anesthetics.

2.6.1.2 Commonly Used Local Anesthetics

The concentration and duration of action vary between local anesthetics. Spinal injection of local anesthetic into the epidural space results in rapid systemic absorption and concentration.

Lidocaine

Lidocaine was the first amino amide type drug widely used for local anesthesia. This agent has a short time to onset (0.5–15 min) and a brief duration (0.5–3 h). The typical concentration is 0.5–2%, and 1% lidocaine contains 1000 mg of lidocaine in 100 mL of fluid (10 mg/mL). The recommended maximum dose of lidocaine is 500 mg [47].

Bupivacaine

Bupivacaine takes effect more slowly (5–20 min) and lasts longer (2–5 h) than lidocaine. The usual concentration is 0.25–0.5% for epidural analgesia and peripheral nerve blocks, as this concentration can induce anesthesia while minimizing the risk of a motor block. The maximum dose of bupivacaine is 80 mg (16 mL of 0.5% solution) intravenously and 225 mg for extravascular sites.

Ropivacaine

Ropivacaine is a long-acting amide local anesthetic agent. Ropivacaine is less lipophilic than bupivacaine, resulting in decreased penetration of large myelinated motor nerves [48]. Ropivacaine's low lipophilicity also leads to low central nervous system toxicity and an increased degree of motor and sensory differentiation. Therefore, ropivacaine is unlikely to cause cardiorespiratory instability, and it allows the selective blockade of nociceptors. The usual concentration is 0.25–0.75% for peripheral nerve and epidural blocks. The ropivacaine has two-thirds the potency of bupivacaine when used for a sensory block.

2.6.1.3 Toxicity

Accidental intravascular administration of local anesthetics may cause central nervous system and cardiopulmonary complications, including nausea, confusion, convulsions, respiratory arrest, and cardiodepression. Frequently, aspiration or identification of vascular uptake using real-time contrast imaging can reduce these adverse effects of local anesthetics during spinal interventions. A brief conversation with the patient or the identification of toxicity symptoms during the procedure may reduce the incidence of significant complications of IV injection of local anesthetic.

2.6.2 Steroids

2.6.2.1 Mechanism of Action

The anabolic effect of corticosteroids effectively reduces inflammation resulting in pain relief. Corticosteroids decrease inflammation by modulating lymphocytes, inhibiting prostaglandin synthesis, blocking immune complex deposition, and reducing capillary permeability [49, 50]. However, in spite of the anti-inflammatory effects of steroids, their role in chronic degenerative disease is controversial. Recently, investigators have reported the therapeutic effect of local anesthetic epidural injection for spinal disease [51]. Therefore, the indications for and frequency of interventions using steroids should be based on the pathophysiology of the disease.

2.6.2.2 Adverse Reactions

Corticosteroids should be used with care as they are associated with adverse reactions. The use of steroids can produce transient flare-up pain for 24–48 h. In patients with diabetes, a steroid injection may increase the blood glucose level for several days after the procedure. Steroids can also cause mild symptoms, including facial flushing, hiccups, insomnia, and mood swings [52–54]. Further, ESIs can produce adhesive arachnoiditis, meningitis, and epidural lipomatosis [55, 56]. Prolonged steroid use can cause osteoporosis, increased susceptibility to infection, osteonecrosis, muscle weakness, cataract, and Cushing syndrome.

2.6.2.3 Spinal Steroid Injections

Some interventionists have reported particulate steroid emboli associated with cervical spinal interventions. Therefore, the risk of steroid emboli should be weighed against the benefits of intervention when considering a spine pain management procedure. A particulate steroid can agglutinate red blood cells sufficiently to block a blood vessel [57]. Non-particulate steroid does not have this property, although the risk of an embolic event is not entirely absent. Moreover, the pain control outcomes after particulate steroid injection are not superior to the results of non-particulate steroid injection [58].

The preservative excipients (PE) can cause neurotoxicity and hypersensitivity during a spinal intervention [59]. Therefore, preservative-free dexamethasone is recommended for transforaminal ESIs (TFESIs) [60]. However, neurotoxicity for the PE benzyl alcohol has never been reported in humans. Moreover, benzyl alcohol hypersensitivity is relatively rare. Therefore, although preservative-free dexamethasone is recommended for spinal interventions, dexamethasone containing PE benzyl alcohol can be a reasonable alternative. In the absence of non-particulate steroids, a particulate steroid can be used for lumbar TFESIs, although its use is not without risk. The use of a particulate steroid is considered relatively safe in caudal and interlaminar procedures, and there is no evidence of any vascular accident associated with interlaminar and caudal particulate steroid injection. Therefore, while the use of non-particulate steroids is recommended whenever possible, particulate steroids can be used in interlaminar and caudal injection if necessary.

References

1. Mihaylov R, Balasubramanian S, Vasu T. Drugs, equipment, and basic principles of spinal interventions. In: Simpson K, editor. Spinal interventions in pain management. New York: Oxford University Press; 2012. p. 23.
2. Chan D, Downing D, Keough CE, Saad WA, Annamalai G, d'Othee BJ, et al. Joint practice guideline for sterile technique during vascular and interventional radiology procedures: from the Society of Interventional Radiology, association of perioperative registered nurses, and Association for Radiologic and Imaging Nursing, for the Society of Interventional Radiology [corrected] standards of practice committee, and endorsed by the cardiovascular interventional radiological Society of Europe and the Canadian interventional radiology association. J Vasc Interv Radiol. 2012;23:1603–12.
3. Kim DH, Choi G, Lee SH. Endoscopic spine surgery. New York: Thieme; 2018.
4. Gupta A. Interventional pain medicine. New York: Oxford University Press; 2012.
5. Manchikanti L, Kaye AD, Falco FJ, Hirsch JA. Essentials of interventional techniques in managing chronic pain. Springer. 2018;
6. Chierichini A, Santoprete S, Frassanito L. Anesthesia and perioperative care in MISS. Minimally invasive surgery of the lumbar spine. Springer; 2014. p. 1–19.
7. Raj PP, Erdine S. Pain-relieving procedures: the illustrated guide. Wiley; 2012.
8. Manchikanti L, Singh V, Pampati V, Boswell MV, Benyamin RM, Hirsch JA. Description of documentation in the management of chronic spinal pain. Pain Physician. 2009;12:E199–224.
9. Manchikanti L, Abdi S, Atluri S, Benyamin RM, Boswell MV, Buenaventura RM, et al. An update of comprehensive evidence-based guidelines for interventional techniques in chronic spinal pain. Part II: guidance and recommendations. Pain Physician. 2013;16(2 Suppl):S49–283.
10. Bogduk N, Aprill C, Dreyfuss P. International spine intervention society practice guidelines for spinal diagnostic and treatment procedures. San Francisco; 2004.
11. Zacharoff KL, Pujol LM, Corsini E. PainEDU.org manual: a pocket guide to pain management. 4th ed. Waltham: Inflexxion; 2010. p. 51–60.
12. Cordner HJ. Patient evaluation and criteria for procedure selection. In: Mathis JM, Golovac S, editors. Image-guided spine interventions. New York: Springer; 2010. p. 39–55.
13. Braddom RL. Physical medicine and rehabilitation e-book. Philadelphia: Elsevier Health Sciences; 2010.
14. van Tulder M, Becker A, Bekkering T, Breen A, del Real MT, Hutchinson A, et al. European guidelines for the management of acute nonspecific low back pain in primary care. Eur Spine J. 2006;15(Suppl 2):S169–91.

15. Devereaux MW. Anatomy and examination of the spine. Neurol Clin. 2007;25:331–51.
16. General Medical Council. Consent: patients and doctors making decisions together. 2008. https://www.gmc-uk.org/-/media/documents/Consent___English_0617.pdf_48903482.pdf. Accessed Day Month (abbreviated form) Year.
17. Gonzalez P, Laker SR, Sullivan W, Harwood JEF, Akuthota V. The effects of epidural betamethasone on blood glucose in patients with diabetes mellitus. PM R. 2009;1:340–5.
18. American Society of Anesthesiologists Task Force on Sedation and Analgesia by Non-Anesthesiologists. Practice guidelines for sedation and analgesia by non-anesthesiologists. Anesthesiology. 2002;96:1004–17.
19. Knape JT, Adriaensen H, van Aken H, Blunnie WP, Carlsson C, Dupont M, et al. Guidelines for sedation and/or analgesia by non-anaesthesiology doctors. Eur J Anaesthesiol. 2007;24:563–7.
20. Warner MA. Practice guidelines for preoperative fasting and the use of pharmacologic agents to reduce the risk of pulmonary aspiration: application to healthy patients undergoing elective procedures. Anesthesiology. 1990;90:896–905.
21. Miller RD. Miller's anesthesia. __ ed. Philadelphia: Elsevier/Saunders; 2015.
22. Katzung BG. Basic & clinical pharmacology. __ ed. New York: Lange Medical Books/McGraw-Hill; 2001.
23. Ward A, Watson J, Wood P, Dunne C, Kerr D. Glucocorticoid epidural for sciatica: metabolic and endocrine sequelae. Rheumatology (Oxford). 2002;41:68–71.
24. Maillefert JF, Aho S, Huguenin MC, Chatard C, Peere T, Marquignon MF, et al. Systemic effects of epidural dexamethasone injections. Rev Rhum Engl Ed. 1995;62:429–32.
25. Botwin KP, Gruber RD, Bouchlas CG, Torres-Ramos FM, Freeman TL, Slaten WK. Complications of fluoroscopically guided transforaminal lumbar epidural injections. Arch Phys Med Rehabil. 2000;81:1045–50.
26. Olsen MA, Nepple JJ, Riew KD, Lenke LG, Bridwell KH, Mayfield J, et al. Risk factors for surgical site infection following orthopaedic spinal operations. J Bone Joint Surg Am. 2008;90:62–9.
27. Mackey DC, Carpenter RL, Thompson GE, Brown DL, Bodily MN. Bradycardia and asystole during spinal anesthesia: a report of three cases without morbidity. Anesthesiology. 1989;70:866–8.
28. Rooke GA, Freund PR, Jacobson AF. Hemodynamic response and change in organ blood volume during spinal anesthesia in elderly men with cardiac disease. Anesth Analg. 1997;85:99–105.
29. Leslie K, Myles P, Devereaux P, Williamson E, Rao-Melancini P, Forbes A, et al. Neuraxial block, death and serious cardiovascular morbidity in the POISE trial. Br J Anaesth. 2013;111:382–90.
30. Pöpping DM, Elia N, Marret E, Remy C, Tramèr MR. Protective effects of epidural analgesia on pulmonary complications after abdominal and thoracic surgery: a meta-analysis. Arch Surg. 2008;143:990–9. discussion 1000
31. Carpenter RL, Caplan RA, Brown DL, Stephenson C, Wu R. Incidence and risk factors for side effects of spinal anesthesia. Anesthesiology. 1992;76:906–16.
32. Narouze S, Benzon HT, Provenzano D, Buvanendran A, De Andres J, Deer T, et al. Interventional spine and pain procedures in patients on antiplatelet and anticoagulant medications (second edition): guidelines from the American Society of Regional Anesthesia and Pain Medicine, the European Society of Regional Anaesthesia and Pain Therapy, the American Academy of Pain Medicine, the International Neuromodulation Society, the North American Neuromodulation Society, and the World Institute of Pain. Reg Anesth Pain Med. 2018;43:225–62.
33. Horlocker TT, Wedel DJ, Rowlingson JC, Enneking FK, Kopp SL, Benzon HT, et al. Regional anesthesia in the patient receiving antithrombotic or thrombolytic therapy: American Society of Regional Anesthesia and Pain Medicine evidence-based guidelines (third edition). Reg Anesth Pain Med. 2010;35:64–101.
34. Gogarten W, Vandermeulen E, Van Aken H, Kozek S, Llau JV, Samama CM. Regional anaesthesia and antithrombotic agents: recommendations of the European Society of Anaesthesiology. Eur J Anaesthesiol. 2010;27:999–1015.
35. Breivik H, Bang U, Jalonen J, Vigfússon G, Alahuhta S, Lagerkranser M. Nordic guidelines for neuraxial blocks in disturbed haemostasis from the Scandinavian society of Anaesthesiology and intensive care medicine. Acta Anaesthesiol Scand. 2010;54:16–41.
36. Zisman E, Erport A, Kohanovsky E, Ballagulah M, Cassel A, Quitt M, et al. Platelet function recovery after cessation of aspirin: preliminary study of volunteers and surgical patients. Eur J Anaesthesiol. 2010;27:617–23.
37. O'Gara PT, Kushner FG, Ascheim DD, Casey DE Jr, Chung MK, de Lemos JA, et al. 2013 ACCF/AHA guideline for the management of ST-elevation myocardial infarction: executive summary: a report of the American College of Cardiology Foundation/American Heart Association task force on practice guidelines. J Am Coll Cardiol. 2013;61:485–510.
38. Benzon HT, Fragen R, Benzon HA, Savage J, Robinson J, Puri L. Clopidogrel and neuraxial block: the role of the PFA II and P2Y12 assays. Reg Anesth Pain Med. 2010;35:115.
39. Conway R, O'Shea FD, Cunnane G, Doran MF. Safety of joint and soft tissue injections in patients on warfarin anticoagulation. Clin Rheumatol. 2013;32:1811–4.
40. Meng H, Fei Q, Wang B, Yang Y, Li D, Li J, et al. Epidural injections with or without steroids in managing chronic low back pain secondary to lumbar spinal stenosis: a meta-analysis of 13 randomized controlled trials. Drug Des Devel Ther. 2015;9:4657–67.
41. Manchikanti L, Singh V, Falco FJ, Cash KA, Pampati V, Fellows B. The role of thoracic medial branch blocks in managing chronic mid and upper back pain: a randomized, double-blind, active-control

trial with a 2-year followup. Anesthesiol Res Pract. 2012;2012:585806.
42. Eggleston ST, Lush LW. Understanding allergic reactions to local anesthetics. Ann Pharmacother. 1996;30:851–7.
43. Speca SJ, Boynes SG, Cuddy MA. Allergic reactions to local anesthetic formulations. Dent Clin N Am. 2010;54:655–64.
44. Becker DE, Reed KL. Essentials of local anesthetic pharmacology. Anesth Prog. 2006;53:98–108; quiz 9-10.
45. DiFazio CA, Carron H, Grosslight KR, Moscicki JC, Bolding WR, Johns RA. Comparison of pH-adjusted lidocaine solutions for epidural anesthesia. Anesth Analg. 1986;65:760–4.
46. Cummins TR. Setting up for the block: the mechanism underlying lidocaine's use-dependent inhibition of sodium channels. J Physiol. 2007;582(Pt 1):11.
47. Rosenberg PH, Veering BT, Urmey WF. Maximum recommended doses of local anesthetics: a multifactorial concept. Reg Anesth Pain Med. 2004;29:564–75.
48. Kuthiala G, Chaudhary G. Ropivacaine: a review of its pharmacology and clinical use. Indian J Anaesth. 2011;55:104–10.
49. Peters WP, Holland JF, Senn H, Rhomberg W, Banerjee T. Corticosteroid administration and localized leukocyte mobilization in man. N Engl J Med. 1972;286:342–5.
50. Schayer RW. Induced synthesis of histamine, microcirculatory regulation and the mechanism of action of the adrenal glucocorticoid hormones. Prog Allergy. 1963;7:187–212.
51. MacMahon PJ, Eustace SJ, Kavanagh EC. Injectable corticosteroid and local anesthetic preparations: a review for radiologists. Radiology. 2009;252:647–61.
52. Everett CR, Baskin MN, Speech D, Novoseletsky D, Patel R. Flushing as a side effect following lumbar transforaminal epidural steroid injection. Pain Physician. 2004;7:427–9.
53. Kaydu A, Kılıç ET, Gökçek E, Akdemir MS. Unexpected complication after caudal epidural steroid injection: hiccup. Anesth Essays Res. 2017;11:776–7.
54. Plastaras C, McCormick ZL, Garvan C, Macron D, Joshi A, Chimes G, et al. Adverse events associated with fluoroscopically guided lumbosacral transforaminal epidural steroid injections. Spine J. 2015;15:2157–65.
55. Nelson DA. Intraspinal therapy using methylprednisolone acetate. Twenty-three years of clinical controversy. Spine (Phila Pa 1976). 1993;18:278–86.
56. McCullen GM, Spurling GR, Webster JS. Epidural lipomatosis complicating lumbar steroid injections. J Spinal Disord. 1999;12:526–9.
57. Derby R, Lee SH, Date ES, Lee JH, Lee CH. Size and aggregation of corticosteroids used for epidural injections. Pain Med. 2008;9:227–34.
58. Mehta P, Syrop I, Singh JR, Kirschner J. Systematic review of the efficacy of particulate versus nonparticulate corticosteroids in epidural injections. PM R. 2017;9:502–12.
59. Van Boxem K, Rijsdijk M, Hans G, de Jong J, Kallewaard JW, Vissers K, et al. Safe use of epidural corticosteroid injections: recommendations of the WIP Benelux work group. Pain Pract. 2019;19:61–92.
60. Duszynski B. Spine intervention society position statement on best practices for epidural steroid injections in the setting of a preservative-free dexamethasone shortage. Pain Med. 2019;20:1277–80.

3 Epidural Approaches: Transforaminal, Interlaminar, and Caudal

Jung Hwan Lee

3.1 Introduction

Epidural injections (EIs) are conducted to treat axial back or radicular pain secondary to disc herniation, stenosis, and other spinal pathologies [1]. Axial back or radicular pain is caused by not only a mechanical component provided by protruded disc or stenosis but also chemical inflammation, which is developed by a reaction between inflammatory mediator and nucleus pulposus materials epidurally released through torn annulus. The EIs of medications, including steroids and local anesthetics, lead to pain reduction by eliminating inflammatory mediators and blocking the conduction of nociceptive stimuli in the epidural space. EIs are conducted through several routes, including the interlaminar (ILEI), transforaminal (TFEI), and caudal approaches (CEI, used only to treat lumbosacral pathology).

The term "selective nerve root block" (SNRB) is sometimes used interchangeably with TFEI. However, an SNRB delivers a small amount of injectate alongside the target spinal nerve, while TFEI delivers a relatively large amount of medication to the epidural space as well as the nerve root. SNRBs are only used to diagnose the pain source and are especially useful in identification of the symptomatic level in patients with multi-level spinal pathology before determining the treatment target when clinical, electrodiagnostic, and radiological findings are equivocal or contradictory.

3.2 Cervical Spine

3.2.1 Anatomical Considerations

Seven cervical vertebral bodies with eight cervical nerve roots existed. The first cervical nerve root is placed between the occiput and C1 vertebra is called the C1 nerve root. The C2 nerve root exits between the C1 and C2 vertebrae, and the subsequent nerve roots are numbered for the number of vertebrae located below. Each cervical nerve root exits from the lower and posterior half of the neural foramen angled approximately 45° anterolaterally and 10° downward.

The understanding of vascular structures around the neural foramina is crucial for the safe and effective performance of TFEI in the cervical spine. The vertebral artery is located immediately ventral and medial to the exiting nerve root. Radicular or segmental medullary arteries, branches of the ascending cervical, deep cervical, and vertebral arteries, traverse the neural foramina, feed the exiting spinal nerve roots, pass through the dura, and anastomose with the anterior and posterior spinal arteries (Fig. 3.1). Therefore, during TFEI, the needle is usually

J. H. Lee (✉)
Namdarun Rehabilitation Clinic,
Yongin-si, Republic of Korea

S.-H. Lee (ed.), *Minimally Invasive Spine Interventions*,
https://doi.org/10.1007/978-981-16-9547-6_3

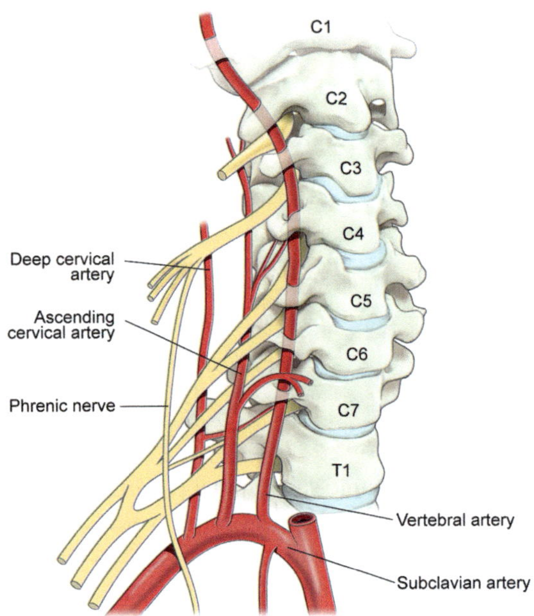

Fig. 3.1 The radicular arteries originate from the ascending cervical, deep cervical, and vertebral arteries and traverse the neural foramina

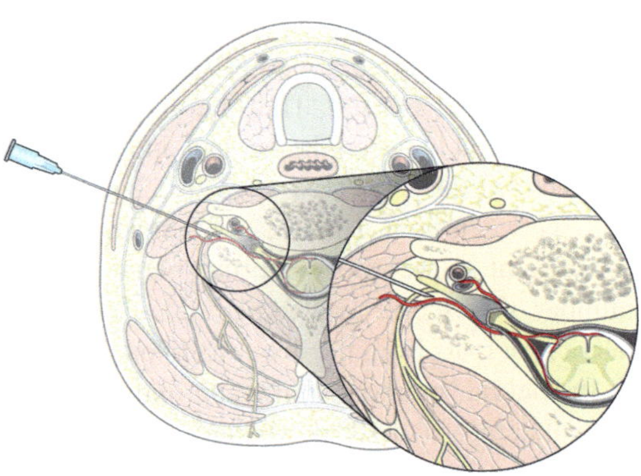

Fig. 3.2 The needle should be advanced over the dorsal part of the neural foramen to avoid penetrating the vertebral artery and the radicular arteries passing through the neural foramina

advanced over the posterior part of the neural foramen to avoid penetrating the vertebral artery (Fig. 3.2). However, according to Huntoon et al.'s cadaveric study, 22% of vessels from the ascending and deep cervical arteries existed within 2 mm of the needle trajectory using the posterior foraminal approach to cervical TFEI and could potentially be cannulated [2]. Therefore, the operator must carefully identify and avoid anatomic variants of radicular arteries, as penetration or occlusion of arterial branches that supply the cervical spinal cord or brainstem produces major adverse events [3].

3.2.2 Techniques

3.2.2.1 Interlaminar Approach

Before beginning a cervical ILEI, the patient is placed in a prone position with neck flexion. An anteroposterior (AP) view of the patient's cervical spine is obtained by C-arm fluoroscopy, and the needle target is determined. Typically, the C6–C7 or C7–T1 interlaminar space is selected as the target because this area has a relatively wide dorsal epidural space, which allows safe and effective drug delivery to the epidural space. The ideal visualization of the aperture of the interlaminar space is usually obtained by tilting the fluoroscope caudally. The skin over the needle entry site is draped under sterile conditions and anesthetized using 1 mL of local anesthetic.

A 22-gauge Tuohy needle is advanced under intermittent fluoroscopic guidance utilizing either the contralateral oblique (CLO) or lateral image to identify the needle depth. The needle is advanced until it touches the inferior lamina to prevent the needle from advancing too deeply and penetrating the dura. The needle is then adjusted into cranial direction and then serially advanced by less than a millimeter per movement using the loss-of-resistance technique to detect the ligamentum flavum and prevent dural penetration; using this method the operator detects a loss of resistance when the needle is inserted into the epidural space. Contrast is injected to confirm the epidural placement of the needle, demonstrated by the characteristic epidural contrast dispersal pattern (Fig. 3.3). At this point, approximately 4–6 mL of combined local anesthetic and steroid is injected into the epidural space.

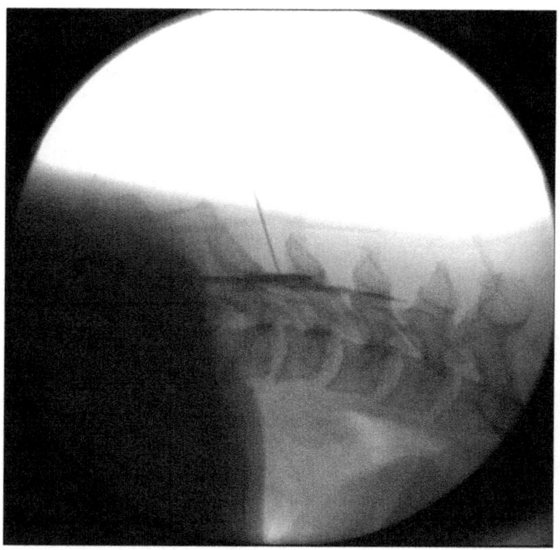

Fig. 3.3 C-arm fluoroscopy (lateral view) shows contrast spreading into the dorsal epidural space during cervical interlaminar epidural injection

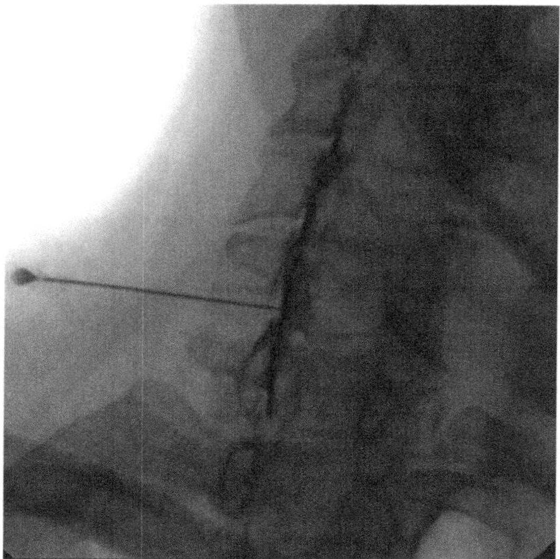

Fig. 3.4 This contralateral oblique view clearly shows the ventral lamina line and facilitates the determination of the appropriate needle depth for a paramedian approach

Contralateral Oblique View
When the needle is located at or near the midline, lateral fluoroscopic views can determine the depth of insertion based on the relationship between the needle and the lamina silhouette. If the needle is located lateral to the midline, the lateral view may magnify the depth of needle insertion. This problem can be prevented using the CLO view, in which the beam of the fluoroscope is directed parallel to the elliptical superior and inferior laminae and the ventral laminar line where the needle tip is placed. The CLO view more clearly visualizes these structures and assesses needle depth accurately, especially when a paramedian ILEI is performed [3] (Fig 3.4). According to Park et al.'s study, when the needle tip is placed within a spinous process, a CLO view oriented 60° from a vertical line through the spinous process is superior to other angles for assessing the epidural space. When the needle tip is placed within the lamina lateral to the spinous processes, a CLO view at 50° is most appropriate (Fig. 3.5) [4].

3.2.2.2 Transforaminal Approach

The patient is placed in the supine position on the table with a bolster placed beneath the shoulder to extend the head slightly. An AP fluoroscopic view is obtained to identify the bony anatomy related to the injection target that was established based on the clinical and radiological evaluations. Then the fluoroscope is rotated obliquely to the ipsilateral side by approximately 40°–50° to supply the best view of the selected neural foramen. The skin directly over the posterior half of the target neuroforamen is draped using sterile technique and anesthetized with a local anesthetic.

A 25-gauge spinal needle is advanced to the division between the middle and lower thirds of the superior articular process (SAP) that form the posterior border of the neural foramen using a tunnel vision technique; this method entails inserting the needle parallel to the fluoroscopic beam, which appears as a single radiopaque dot superimposed over the target. After contacting the target, the needle is slightly redirected anteriorly and advanced into the neural foramen. The needle is moved forward to the midpoint of the medial and lateral borders of the articular pillars in an AP view. The needle should not be administered beyond this point to prevent accidental damage to the vertebral artery and nerve root. At that point, 0.5 mL of contrast media is injected under real-time fluoroscopic view to demonstrate contrast spread along the nerve root and epidural

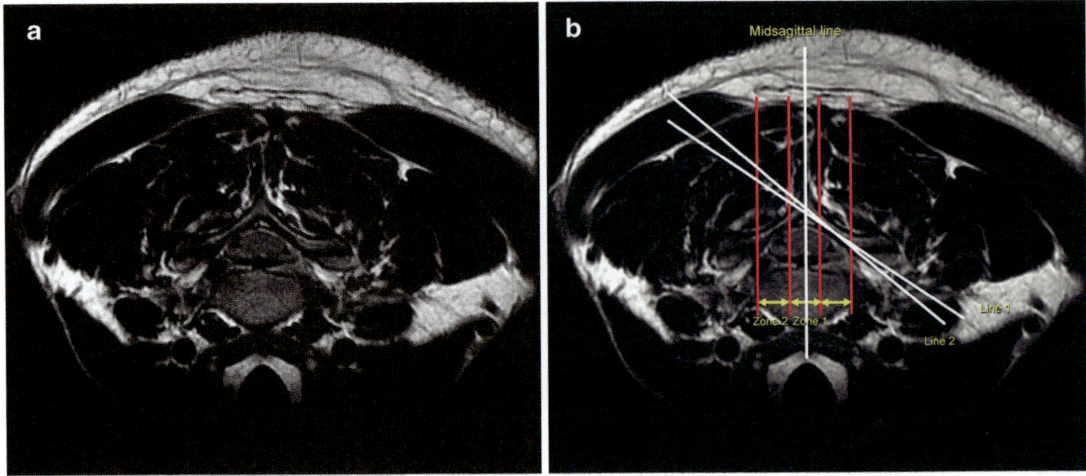

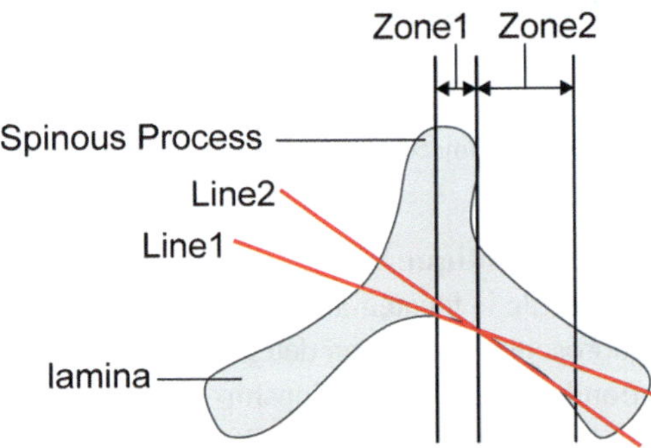

Fig. 3.5 The appropriate angle of contralateral oblique (CLO) view lines during C-arm fluoroscopy according to needle placement (when the needle tip is placed within a spinous process [Zone 1], Line 1 oriented at 60° from a vertical line through the spinous process is optimal for assessing the epidural space, while Line 2 at 50° is optimal when the needle tip is placed within the lamina lateral to the spinous process [Zone 2])

space and confirm the absence of vascular or intrathecal contrast flow (Fig. 3.6). A maximum of 2 mL of a mixed injectate of local anesthetic and steroid is slowly injected.

3.2.3 Complications

Minor adverse events during cervical EI include non-specific headache, nausea and vomiting, vasovagal reaction, facial flushing, transient lightheadedness, and transient paresthesia. Inadvertent intra-arterial penetration into the vertebral artery or radiculomedullary arteries during TFEI can produce vascular occlusion and subsequent spinal cord or brainstem embolic infarction, especially when a particulate steroid is injected and forms intravascular aggregates. Intra-arterial injection of local anesthetics can induce seizures, cardiopulmonary arrest, or death. Further, a direct spinal cord injury or epidural hematoma can occur during ILEI [5].

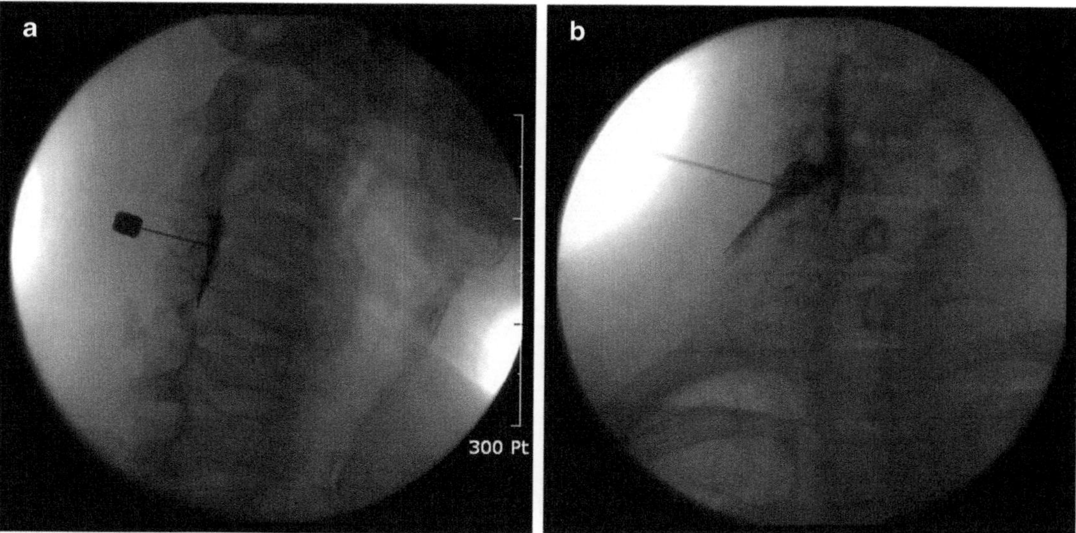

Fig. 3.6 Cervical transforaminal epidural injection: fluoroscopic images show contrast spreading into the epidural space in oblique (**a**) and anteroposterior (**b**) views

3.3 Thoracic Spine

3.3.1 Anatomical Considerations

Each thoracic spinal nerve exits from the posterior, upper half of its corresponding intervertebral foramen; for example, the T2 spinal nerve exits from the neural foramen between the T2 and T3 vertebrae. The anatomy of the upper thoracic levels (T1–T8), including the shape of the vertebral lamina, the narrow spaces between ribs, and the wide bases of the transverse processes, makes it difficult to identify the neural foramina. Consequently, the accurate placement of a straight needle for the TFEI and SNRB procedures is also difficult. The use of a curved needle makes accurate cannula positioning easy.

During thoracic ESI, the major anatomical considerations are the proximity to intrathoracic organs, such as the lung, pleura, mediastinum, and heart, and the presence of the ribs protecting these structures. Each rib contacts the inferior part of the neural foramen at the lateral margin of the transverse process of the inferior vertebral body. This anatomical relationship between the ribs and vertebrae allows physicians to use a rib as a depth gauge that prevents an intrathoracic organ puncture and to guide the needle into the intervertebral foramen.

Further, during lower thoracic TFEI or SNRB, the operator should avoid penetrating the artery of Adamkiewicz, the largest anterior radicular artery that supplies the thoracic spinal cord below T9. Due to its large size, this artery is at risk of a puncture during TFESI or SNRB, and, as it supplies a broad area, its thrombotic occlusion can result in devastating complications, including lower-limb paraplegia from spinal cord infarction.

3.3.2 Techniques

3.3.2.1 Interlaminar Approach

Thoracic ILEIs are typically performed using a paramedian approach. The significant downward angulation of the overlapping thoracic spinous processes makes it difficult to perform a median (midline) approach, particularly at the mid- to upper thoracic levels.

An AP view is obtained using C-arm fluoroscopy; a slight cephalic or caudal tilt is needed to visualize the interlaminar space maximally. The needle insertion site is identified in the parame-

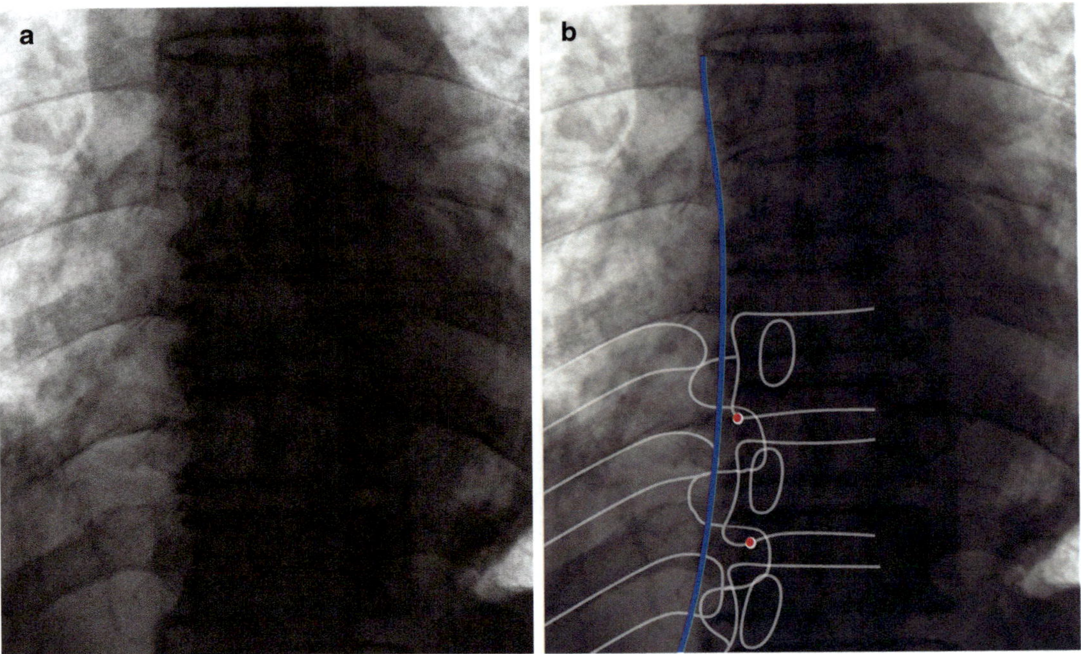

Fig. 3.7 The target points for a thoracic transforaminal epidural injection (*red dots*) and the mediastinal line (*dotted line*) *P*, pedicle; *R*, rib

dian area of the symptomatic interlaminar space. After that, the fluoroscope is rotated ipsilaterally approximately 5° to obtain a trajectory view, and a 22-gauge Tuohy needle is advanced under direct fluoroscopic vision. Then, the needle depth is determined using the CLO view.

The loss-of-resistance technique is used to penetrate the ligamentum flavum and place the needle into the epidural space. Then, contrast is injected to confirm the epidural placement of the needle, demonstrated by the characteristic epidural contrast dispersal pattern. At this point, a combination of local anesthetic and steroid (approximately 4–6 mL) is injected into the epidural space.

3.3.2.2 Transforaminal Approach

The patient is placed in the prone position. An AP view is obtained via C-arm fluoroscopy, and then the fluoroscope is rotated approximately 10–20° ipsilaterally to the symptomatic side to obtain a trajectory view. The needle insertion site is identified at the posterosuperior aspect of the rib near the junction of its medial part and the transverse process of the lower vertebrae (Fig. 3.7). Then, a spinal needle is advanced under direct fluoroscopic vision to contact the posterosuperior aspect of the rib. After that, the needle tip is repositioned cranially over the lateral border of the transverse process and advanced into the neural foramen. This approach allows the operator to avoid penetrating the intrathoracic organs with the needle.

The needle tip is then positioned at the posterior margin of the neural foramen and the anterior edge of the superior articular process in the lateral view and the 6-o'clock position of the pedicle in the AP view. The needle is advanced anteriorly into the middle or posterior region of the neural foramen. Positioning the needle in this fashion helps prevent intravascular administration of the injectate because the vascular plexus typically resides along the posterior margin of the vertebral body. Contrast media is injected, and its spread into the epidural space is verified. Then, a mixture of local anesthetic and steroid is injected.

3.3.3 Complications

Major adverse effects or complications are rare. Botwin et al. found that complications included injection site pain (7.7%), facial flushing (5.1%), transient non-positional headache (2.6%), insomnia the night of the injection (2.6%), and fever the night of the procedure (2.6%) in 21 patients who received 39 injections [6].

3.4 Lumbosacral Spine

3.4.1 Anatomical Considerations

The lumbar nerves travel inferiorly under the pedicle and along the superior portion of the neural foramen at varying angles. Compared with the lower nerve roots, the upper lumbar roots are located inferiorly in the neural foramen and extend outward closer to the disc level; the lower the lumbar nerve root, the more superior the nerve's position within the neural foramen (Fig. 3.8). The "safe triangle" is the typical site of approach for supraneural TFEI or SNRB procedures. This triangle is defined as the area between the horizontal base of the pedicle, the lateral border of the vertebral body, and the connecting diagonal nerve root. Kambin's triangle is another site of approach for infraneural or retrodiscal TFEI.

Some physicians prefer this approach over the classical supraneural TFEI because they believe that infraneural procedures are theoretically safer, as the probability of encountering the radicular artery in the inferior foramen may be less likely. Kambin's triangle is defined as the area between the inferior portion of the nerve root, the anterior aspect of the SAP, and the superior endplate of the inferior vertebral body.

A thorough understanding of sacral anatomy is necessary for the safe and precise performance of the sacral TFEI and SNRB procedures. The sacrum has a curved wedge shape and consists of five fused sacral vertebrae. Each of four pairs of sacral foramina is formed by its upper

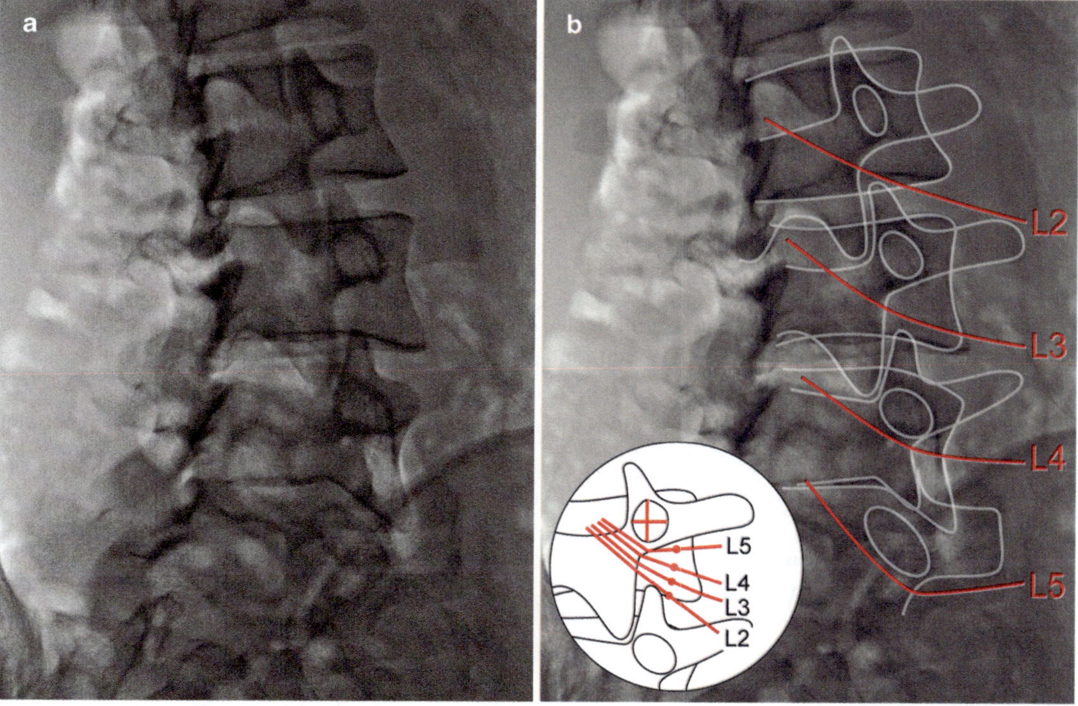

Fig. 3.8 The location of lumbar nerve roots exiting the neural foramina: within the neural foramina, the upper lumbar roots descend more steeply, and the lower lumbar nerve roots occupy a superior position; L, lumbar

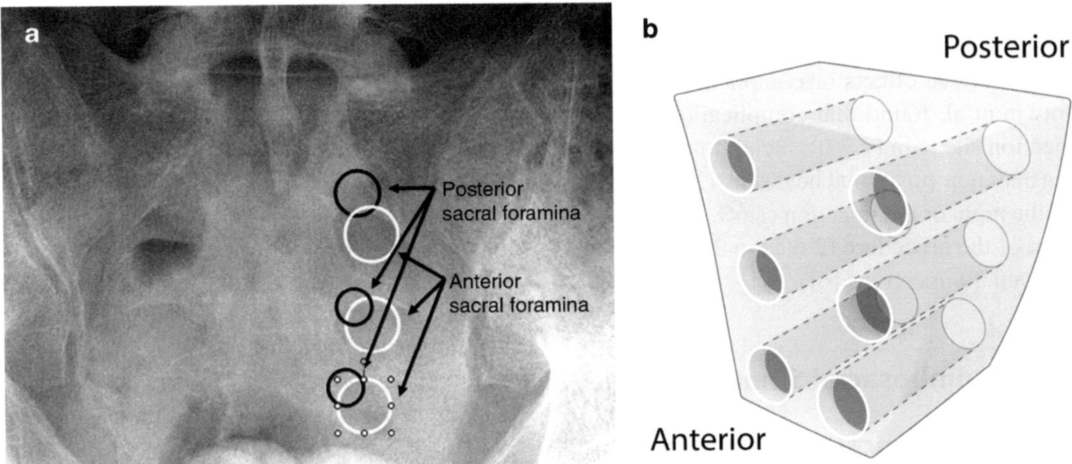

Fig. 3.9 An X-ray (anteroposterior view) reveals anterior and posterior neural foramina simultaneously: the posterior sacral foramina appear as small circles, whereas the anterior foramina have a curvilinear shape

and lower fused sacral vertebrae, and the pelvic and dorsal sacral surfaces have anterior and posterior sacral foramina, respectively. These foramina act as conduits for the anterior and posterior sacral nerve roots and accompanying vessels. On an X-ray, the anterior and posterior sacral foramina overlap in the AP view. Although they are frequently difficult to distinguish, the posterior foramina appear as small circles, while the anterior foramina have a curvilinear shape (Fig. 3.9).

3.4.2 Techniques

3.4.2.1 Interlaminar Approach

The patient is placed in the prone or lateral decubitus position, and an AP image with or without cephalad tilt is obtained. The target is the superior interlaminar space on the symptomatic side at the pathologic level or one caudal level. A 22-gauge Tuohy needle is introduced slightly caudal to the target and directed cephalad toward the paramedian interlaminar space. The needle should enter the site at an oblique rather than a perpendicular angle to decrease the risk of dural puncture.

With the approach described here, the needle is placed using a trajectory view and advanced under the guidance of multiplanar imaging. The needle's depth is confirmed using the CLO or lateral view, or both, to visualize the ventral interlaminar or spinolaminar line. The CLO view is preferable to the lateral view as a guide for needle advancement to the interlaminar space. A subtle change in resistance marks ligamentum flavum penetration, and the loss of resistance to air or saline injection is noted upon entering the epidural space. Correct epidural needle placement is confirmed by injecting approximately 1.0 to 2.0 ml of contrast media under AP and lateral C-arm fluoroscopic views (Fig. 3.10). After confirming that contrast spreads into the epidural space, 5–6 ml of a mixture of local anesthetics and a steroid is introduced.

3.4.2.2 Transforaminal Approaches

Supraneural Approach

The patient is placed in the prone position. The fluoroscope is rotated in the caudal or cephalad direction until the superior endplate of the lower vertebra appears as a straight line, indicating a true AP fluoroscopic view that is aligned in parallel with the superior endplate of the lower vertebra. Then, the fluoroscope is rotated 20° to 30° ipsilaterally toward the symptomatic side until the "Scotty dog" configuration is identified. In this view, the transverse process, pedicle, inferior articular process, and superior articular process appear as a dog's nose, eye, front leg, and ear, respectively. A more oblique view allows a more

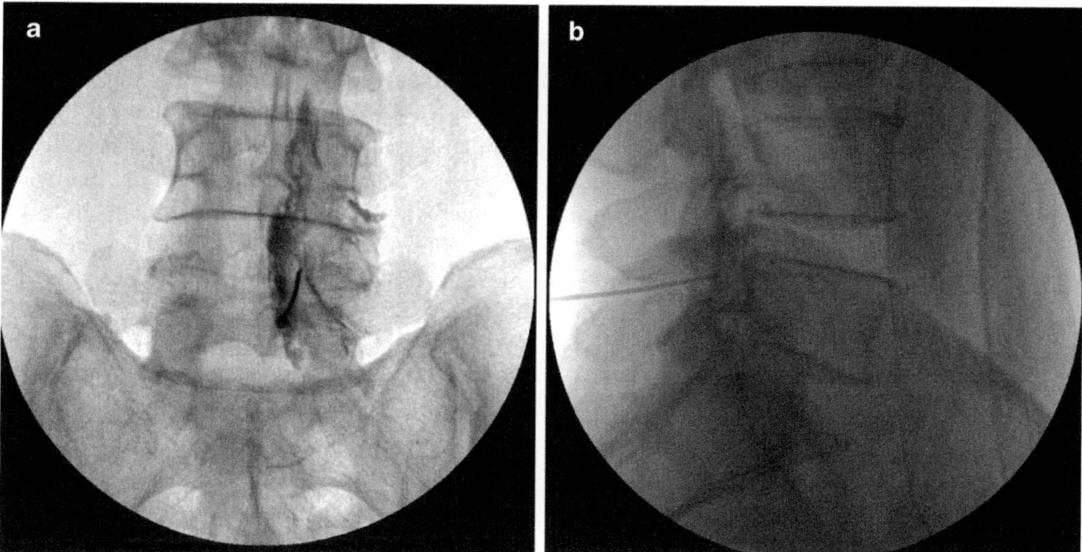

Fig. 3.10 Fluoroscopic images show contrast flowing into the epidural space during lumbar interlaminar epidural injection: anteroposterior (**a**) and lateral (**b**) views

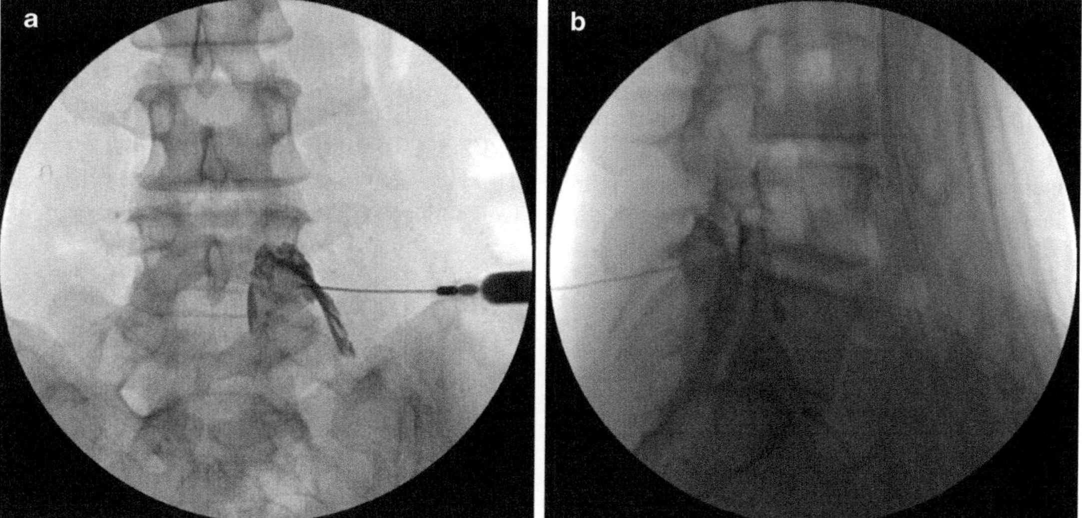

Fig. 3.11 Fluoroscopic images show contrast flowing into the epidural space during lumbar transforaminal epidural injection: oblique (**a**) and lateral (**b**) views

obtuse needle trajectory and a more dorsomedial needle tip placement. This view facilitates the approach to the neural foramen in patients with foraminal stenosis. In contrast, a less oblique view allows a more acute needle trajectory and a more ventral needle tip placement.

The needle is advanced just below the pedicle's 6-o'clock position using a tunnel vision technique under fluoroscopic guidance. The operator should avoid passing the needle medial to the mid-pedicle position in the oblique view to reduce the risk of a dural puncture. Contrast dye is injected to confirm flow within the epidural space without intravascular, intrathecal, or soft tissue flow. A lateral view is also obtained to verify that contrast media is present in the ventral epidural space (Fig. 3.11). Then, a mixture of local anesthetic and steroid is injected.

Infraneural Approach

This alternative method is called the infraneural technique because the needle stays in the lower third of the foramen or "low in the hole." The technique is also described as the retrodiscal or preganglionic approach because the needle is introduced just posterior to the disc's posterior annulus or proximal to the dorsal root ganglion (DRG) of the traversing nerve root. The infraneural technique has the advantage of administering injectate into the epidural space posterior to the targeted disc level as well as along the traversing nerve root. However, it also carries the risk of inadvertent needle penetration into the disc.

The infraneural approach is performed in the same way as the supraneural approach except that the needle target is Kambin's triangle, similar to that of lumbosacral discography. The needle should be placed as low as possible in the lower third of the foramen (Fig. 3.12).

S1 Transforaminal Injection

S1 transforaminal injection is performed through the posterior S1 sacral foramen. It is often difficult to obtain the optimal view of the posterior S1 foramen in the AP fluoroscopic view because the anterior and posterior S1 foramina overlap in this view and are not easily distinguished. Therefore, the fluoroscope is tilted cephalad to separate the foramina and allow visualization of the posterior S1 foramen. In this view, the S1 superior endplate is aligned in parallel with the L5 inferior endplate. If the posterior foramen is still not clearly visible, the fluoroscope should be rotated obliquely to the ipsilateral side by 5° to 10°. This view allows visualization of the S1 pedicle and the superolateral margin of the posterior S1 foramen.

The spinal needle is advanced under fluoroscopy using the tunnel vision technique until it contacts the superolateral margin of the posterior S1 foramen. This step confirms the depth and direction of the needle before it enters the sacral foramen. Then, the needle is advanced until its tip is located 1 to 2 mm anterior to the posterior edge of the sacrum, and a lateral image is obtained to verify that the needle is not advanced through the anterior foramen into the pelvis (Fig. 3.13). Injection of contrast dye under real-time fluoroscopic guidance is necessary to avoid intravascular injection of medication, the risk of which is high due to the numerous vessels in this region.

3.4.2.3 Caudal Approach

The patient is placed in a prone position with legs abducted. After the sacral hiatus is identi-

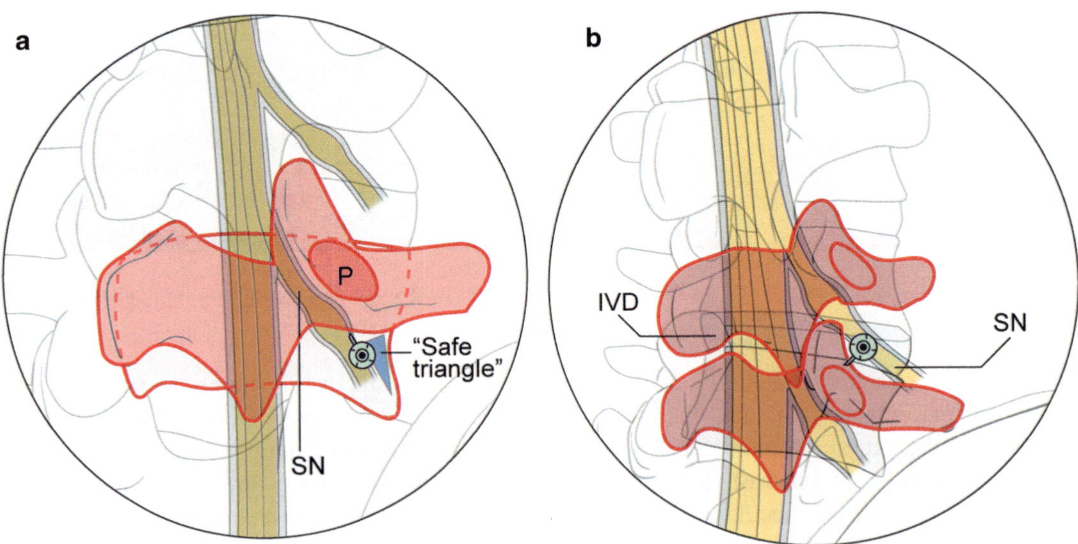

Fig. 3.12 Fluoroscopic images and matched illustrations show the needle position in, and anatomical considerations of, supraneural (**a**) and infraneural (**b**) approaches to lumbosacral transforaminal injection

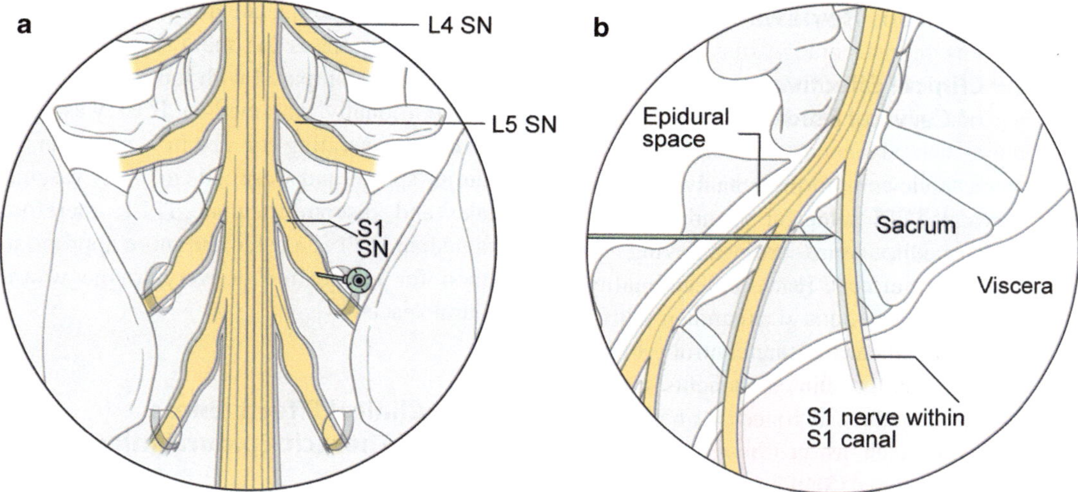

Fig. 3.13 Fluoroscopic contrast images and corresponding illustrations demonstrate the needle position and anatomical considerations during S1 transforaminal injection: anteroposterior (**a**) and lateral (**b**) views

fied, a spinal needle is inserted through the sacral hiatus into the sacrococcygeal ligament at a 45° angle. As the sacrococcygeal ligament is punctured, the operator will feel a "pop," and then the needle is advanced to contact the interior wall of the sacral canal. After that, the needle should be withdrawn slightly and advanced into the sacral canal under fluoroscopic visualization in the lateral view. Contrast media is injected under real-time fluoroscopic view to determine the needle placement and make sure that there is no intravasation or subarachnoid spread (Fig. 3.14). A combination of local anesthetic and steroid (approximately 10–15 ml) is injected.

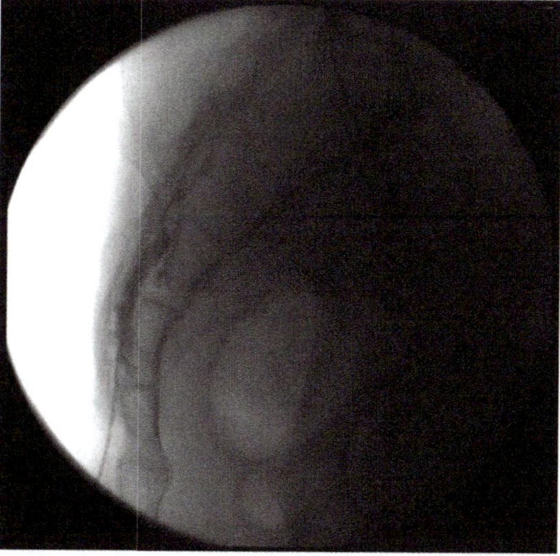

Fig. 3.14 A fluoroscopic image (lateral view) shows contrast flowing into the epidural space after caudal epidural injection

3.4.3 Complications

A lumbar EI can cause a dural puncture, subdural or intravascular injection, spinal cord trauma, intracranial air injection, nerve damage, vascular injury, infection, abscess or hematoma formation, epidural lipomatosis, cerebral vascular or pulmonary embolus, headache, increased ICP, brain damage, death, and adverse steroid effects.

However, contrary to concerns, one study indicated that the continued use of medications associated with a bleeding tendency, such as warfarin, heparin, aspirin, and clopidogrel, did not increase the incidence of clinically relevant epidural hematoma or the aggravation of back or radicular pain [7].

3.5 Previous Reviews

3.5.1 Clinical Effectiveness of Cervical Epidural Injection

Systematic reviews with meta-analysis reported that cervical TFEI achieved meaningful short- and intermediate-term pain-relieving and surgery-sparing effects. However, the quality of evidence is considered low as studies with placebo or active standard of care control groups are lacking. Further, the clinical benefits could be diminished secondary to concerns about serious complications such as death and catastrophic neurological damage [8, 9].

At least one relevant, high-quality randomized controlled trial (RCT) with level II evidence showed that cervical ILEI had clinical benefits in patients with disc herniation, discogenic pain, stenosis, or post-surgery syndrome after a 12–24-month follow-up [10].

3.5.2 Comparison of Cervical Transforaminal and Interlaminar Epidural Injection Approaches

TFEI is reportedly superior to ILEI for the treatment of radiating pain secondary to cervical disc herniation. TFEI resulted in medication placement directly around the affected DRG, whereas in ILEI, injectate delivered to the dorsal epidural space frequently failed to spread to the DRG [11]. Expectedly, compared with ILEI, TFEI achieved better outcomes and a lower incidence of subsequent surgery in patients with radicular arm pain [11, 12].

However, TFEI was not more effective than ILEI for the treatment of axial neck pain as the condition originates mainly in the ventral epidural space. Cervical TFEI is performed in the supine position, and the needle is advanced toward the posterior aspect of the neural foramen to avoid penetration of the vertebral artery. Therefore, TFEI had no advantage over ILEI because, usually, injectate could not be directly administered into the ventral epidural space. The inability to deliver injectate directly into the ventral epidural space is the main disadvantage of cervical TFEI, compared with lumbosacral TFEI [13]. Additionally, paramedian ILEI was more effective in generating contrast flow in the ventral epidural space and resulted in less vascular uptake and discomfort than TFEI; therefore, paramedian ILEI is a safer and more appropriate method for medication delivery to the ventral epidural space [14].

3.5.3 Clinical Effectiveness of Thoracic Epidural Injection

An RCT in patients with mid-thoracic pain secondary to disc herniation or radiculitis and discogenic pain showed that thoracic ILEI led to significant improvement in 71% of the group that received local anesthetic alone and 80% in the group that received a steroid with local anesthetic after 2 years [15].

3.5.4 Clinical Effectiveness of Lumbar Epidural Injection

Five systematic reviews concurred that EI was effective in patients with lumbosacral disc herniation with a high level of evidence [16–20]. Although the evidence supporting short-term clinical effects was strong, the evidence supporting long-term effects was less convincing [17, 20]. There was criticism regarding EI in that its clinical efficacy diminished over time and could not be prolonged. However, the clinical outcomes at long-term follow-up could not be attributed to previous EIs because the pharmacological effects induced by injected drug substantially deteriorated over time [21–23]. Thus, the main goal of EI is to control pain rapidly rather than to provide a lasting effect.

In patients with partial pain reduction after the first EI, those who received repeated EIs at regular 2- to 3-week intervals experienced greater and longer-lasting pain relief than those who underwent repeated injections administered on an irregular, as-needed basis. Further, the latter group required a greater number of EIs, although this difference was not significant. This clinical benefit obtained by repeated injection at regular intervals was also observed in patients with cervical disc herniation and stenosis [24, 25].

3.5.5 Comparison of Three Approaches to Lumbar Epidural Injection

Recent meta-analyses comparing the clinical efficacy of different approaches to lumbar EI showed that TFEI was superior to both ILEI and CEI [26, 27].

Given that axial back and radicular leg pain are mainly originated from sinuvertebral nerves within the ventral epidural space, the nerve root sheath, and the DRG, the main target of drug delivery is the ventral epidural space rather than the dorsal epidural space [28, 29]. Therefore, some physicians prefer TFEI because, with this method, medication is injected directly into the ventral epidural space [30–33], while, with ILEI, medication is administered to the posterior epidural space with the expectation that it will subsequently spread to the ventral space [34–37].

Of ten RCTs that compared TFEI and ILEI, five identified no significant difference in clinical efficacy between the procedures [28, 38–41], four reported that TFEI resulted in significantly better clinical effects during the 3–12-month follow-up [42–45], and one noted that TFEI was more effective in the short term, although this superiority diminished after 2 weeks [46]. Of two non-RCT studies, one revealed no significant difference between the two techniques [47], and the other found that TFEI obtained better clinical efficacy than ILEI [34]. Overall, TFEI showed no inferior or superior clinical results to ILEI for the treatment of patients with pain and functional impairment secondary to lumbar disc herniation.

While some studies showed that TFEI targeted the ventral epidural space more effectively than ILEI [42–44, 48], others showed that ILEI was equally able to deliver medication to the ventral epidural space [39, 49, 50], and the magnitude of ventral epidural spread after ILEI was comparable to that after TFEI [38, 51].

Of four RCTs that compared TFEI and CEI, three demonstrated that TFEI produced better clinical outcomes than CEI during the 6-month follow-up [43–45], and one found that CEI was superior to TFEI [52]. Notably, the latter study used a larger amount of medication (over 30 mL) during CEI than the other three. Of two non-RCTs, one found that TFEI achieved better clinical efficacy than CEI [53], whereas the other indicated no significant difference between the two techniques [47]. Overall, TFEI had no inferior or superior clinical outcomes to CEI for the treatment of patients with pain related to lumbar disc herniation.

3.5.6 Midline Versus Paramedian Approach to Lumbar Interlaminar Epidural Injection

While some physicians prefer a midline approach, others paramedian approach with the belief that ventral drug spread is more reliably accomplished by the paramedian approach in lumbar ILEI [54]. However, studies in both the lumbar and cervical spine revealed no significant difference in treatment effectiveness between the midline and paramedian techniques [54].

3.5.7 Particulate Versus Non-particulate Steroid

Particulated steroids have been regarded as having advantage related to depot effect over non-particulated steroid. However, there have been reports of permanent neurologic complication after cervical TFEI with a particulate agent. Inadvertent intra-arterial (vertebral artery and radiculomedullary arteries) injection of a particulate steroid during cervical TFEI may result in embolic infarction by vascular occlusion. Furthermore, recent comparative clinical outcome research suggests that non-particulate steroids should be considered first-line agents when performing EI because comparisons of particulate and non-particulate corticosteroids showed no between-type difference in pain reduction or functional outcome, and particulate steroids could produce serious complications [55, 56].

References

1. Rivera CE. Lumbar epidural steroid injections. Phys Med Rehabil Clin N Am. 2018;29:73–92.
2. Huntoon MA. Anatomy of the cervical intervertebral foramina: vulnerable arteries and ischemic neurologic injuries after transforaminal epidural injections. Pain. 2005;117:104–11.
3. House LM, Barrette K, Mattie R, McCormick ZL. Cervical epidural steroid injection: techniques and evidence. Phys Med Rehabil Clin N Am. 2018;29:1–17.
4. Park JY, Karm MH, Kim DH, Lee JY, Yun HJ. Optimal angle of contralateral oblique view in cervical interlaminar epidural. 2017;20:E169–75.
5. Candido KD, Knezevic N. Cervical epidural steroid injections for the treatment of cervical spinal (neck) pain. Curr Pain Headache Rep. 2013;17:314.
6. Botwin KP, Baskin M, Rao S. Adverse effects of fluoroscopically guided interlaminar thoracic epidural steroid injections. Am J Phys Med Rehabil. 2006;85:14–23.
7. Park TK, Shin SJ, Lee JH. Effect of drugs associated with bleeding tendency on the complications and outcomes of transforaminal epidural steroid injection. Clin Spine Surg. 2017;30:E104–e10.
8. Conger A, Cushman DM, Speckman RA, Burnham T, Teramoto M, McCormick ZL. The effectiveness of fluoroscopically guided cervical transforaminal epidural steroid injection for the treatment of radicular pain; a systematic review and meta-analysis. Pain Med. 2020;41–54
9. Engel A, King W, MacVicar J. The effectiveness and risks of fluoroscopically guided cervical transforaminal injections of steroids: a systematic review with comprehensive analysis of the published data. Pain Med. 2014;15:386–402.
10. Manchikanti L, Nampiaparampil DE, Candido KD, Bakshi S, Grider JS, Falco FJ, et al. Do cervical epidural injections provide long-term relief in neck and upper extremity pain? A systematic review. Pain Physician. 2015;18:39–60.
11. Huston CW. Cervical epidural steroid injections in the management of cervical radiculitis: interlaminar versus transforaminal. A review. Curr Rev Musculoskelet Med. 2009;2:30–42.
12. Bush K, Hillier S. Outcome of cervical radiculopathy treated with periradicular/epidural corticosteroid injections: a prospective study with independent clinical review. Eur Spine J. 1996;5:319–25.
13. Lee JH, Lee SH. Comparison of clinical efficacy between interlaminar and transforaminal epidural injection in patients with axial pain due to cervical disc herniation. Medicine (Baltimore). 2016;95:e2568.
14. Choi E, Nahm FS, Lee PB. Comparison of contrast flow and clinical effectiveness between a modified paramedian interlaminar approach and transforaminal approach in cervical epidural steroid injection. Br J Anaesth. 2015;115:768–74.
15. Manchikanti L, Cash KA, McManus CD, Pampati V, Benyamin RM. Thoracic interlaminar epidural injections in managing chronic thoracic pain: a randomized, double-blind, controlled trial with a 2-year follow-up. Pain Physician. 2014;17:E327–38.
16. Bhatti AB, Kim S. Role of epidural injections to prevent surgical intervention in patients with chronic sciatica: a systematic review and meta-analysis. Cureus. 2016;8:e723.
17. Manchikanti L, Benyamin RM, Falco FJ, Kaye AD, Hirsch JA. Do epidural injections provide short- and long-term relief for lumbar disc herniation? A systematic review. Clin Orthop Relat Res. 2015;473:1940–56.
18. Kozlov N, Benzon HT, Malik K. Epidural steroid injections: update on efficacy, safety, and newer medications for injection. Minerva Anestesiol. 2015;81:901–9.
19. Bicket MC, Horowitz JM, Benzon HT, Cohen SP. Epidural injections in prevention of surgery for spinal pain: systematic review and meta-analysis of randomized controlled trials. Spine J. 2015;15:348–62.
20. Shamliyan TA, Staal JB, Goldmann D, Sands-Lincoln M. Epidural steroid injections for radicular lumbosacral pain: a systematic review. Phys Med Rehabil Clin N Am. 2014;25:471–89 e1–50.
21. Kennedy DJ, Zheng PZ, Smuck M, McCormick ZL, Huynh L, Schneider BJ. A minimum of 5-year follow-up after lumbar transforaminal epidural steroid injections in patients with lumbar radicular pain due to intervertebral disc herniation. Spine J. 2018;18:29–35.
22. Landa J, Kim Y. Outcomes of interlaminar and transforminal spinal injections. Bull NYU Hosp Jt Dis. 2012;70:6–10.
23. Young IA, Hyman GS, Packia-Raj LN, Cole AJ. The use of lumbar epidural/transforaminal steroids for managing spinal disease. J Am Acad Orthop Surg. 2007;15:228–38.
24. Lee JH, Lee SH. Can repeat injection provide clinical benefit in patients with cervical disc herniation and stenosis when the first epidural injection results only in partial response? Medicine (Baltimore). 2016;95:e4131.
25. Lee JH, Lee SH. Can repeat injection provide clinical benefit in patients with lumbosacral diseases when first epidural injection results only in partial response? Pain Physician. 2016;19:E283–90.
26. Lee JH, Shin KH, Bahk SJ, Lee GJ, Kim DH, Lee CH, et al. Comparison of clinical efficacy of transforami-

nal and caudal epidural steroid injection in lumbar and lumbosacral disc herniation: a systematic review and meta-analysis. Spine J. 2018;18:2343–53.

27. Lee JH, Shin KH, Park SJ, Lee GJ, Lee CH, Kim DH, et al. Comparison of clinical efficacy between transforaminal and interlaminar epidural injections in lumbosacral disc herniation: a systematic review and meta-analysis. Pain Physician. 2018;21:433–48.
28. Lee JH, An JH, Lee SH. Comparison of the effectiveness of interlaminar and bilateral transforaminal epidural steroid injections in treatment of patients with lumbosacral disc herniation and spinal stenosis. Clin J Pain. 2009;25:206–10.
29. McLain RF, Kapural L, Mekhail NA. Epidural steroid therapy for back and leg pain: mechanisms of action and efficacy. Spine J. 2005;5:191–201.
30. Mehta N, Salaria M, Salaria AQ. Comparison of fluoroscopic guided transforaminal epidural injections of steroid and local anaesthetic with conservative management in patients with chronic lumbar radiculopathies. Anesth Essays Res. 2017;11:17–22.
31. Liu J, Zhou H, Lu L, Li X, Jia J, Shi Z, et al. The effectiveness of transforaminal versus caudal routes for epidural steroid injections in managing lumbosacral radicular pain: a systematic review and meta-analysis. Medicine (Baltimore). 2016;95:e3373.
32. Pairuchvej S, Arirachakaran A, Keorochana G, Wattanapaiboon K, Atiprayoon S, Phatthanathitikarn P, et al. The short and midterm outcomes of lumbar transforaminal epidural injection with preganglionic and postganglionic approach in lumbosacral radiculopathy: a systematic review and meta-analysis. Neurosurg Rev. 2018;41:909–16.
33. Lutz GE, Vad VB, Wisneski RJ. Fluoroscopic transforaminal lumbar epidural steroids: an outcome study. Arch Phys Med Rehabil. 1998;79:1362–6.
34. Schaufele MK, Hatch L, Jones W. Interlaminar versus transforaminal epidural injections for the treatment of symptomatic lumbar intervertebral disc herniations. Pain Physician. 2006;9:361–6.
35. Botwin K, Natalicchio J, Brown LA. Epidurography contrast patterns with fluoroscopic guided lumbar transforaminal epidural injections: a prospective evaluation. Pain Physician. 2004;7:211–5.
36. Cooper G, Lutz GE, Boachie-Adjei O, Lin J. Effectiveness of transforaminal epidural steroid injections in patients with degenerative lumbar scoliotic stenosis and radiculopathy. Pain Physician. 2004;7:311–7.
37. Bhatia A, Flamer D, Shah PS, Cohen SP. Transforaminal epidural steroid injections for treating lumbosacral radicular pain from herniated intervertebral discs: a systematic review and meta-analysis. Anesth Analg. 2016;122:857–70.
38. Ghai B, Bansal D, Kay JP, Vadaje KS, Wig J. Transforaminal versus parasagittal interlaminar epidural steroid injection in low back pain with radicular pain: a randomized, double-blind, active-control trial. Pain Physician. 2014;17:277–90.
39. Rados I, Sakic K, Fingler M, Kapural L. Efficacy of interlaminar vs transforaminal epidural steroid injection for the treatment of chronic unilateral radicular pain: prospective, randomized study. Pain Med. 2011;12:1316–21.
40. Hashemi SM, Aryani MR, Momenzadeh S, Razavi SS, Mohseni G, Mohajerani SA, et al. Comparison of transforaminal and parasagittal epidural steroid injections in patients with radicular low back pain. Anesth Pain Med. 2015;5:e26652.
41. Candido KD, Raghavendra MS, Chinthagada M, Badiee S, Trepashko DW. A prospective evaluation of iodinated contrast flow patterns with fluoroscopically guided lumbar epidural steroid injections: the lateral parasagittal interlaminar epidural approach versus the transforaminal epidural approach. Anesth Analg. 2008;106:638–44, table of contents.
42. Rezende R, Jacob Junior C, da Silva CK, de Barcellos ZI, Cardoso IM, Batista Junior JL. Comparison of the efficacy of transforaminal and interlaminar radicular block techniques for treating lumbar disk hernia. Rev Bras Ortop. 2015;50:220–5.
43. Pandey RA. Efficacy of epidural steroid injection in management of lumbar prolapsed intervertebral disc: a comparison of caudal, transforaminal and interlaminar routes. J Clin Diagn Res. 2016;10:RC05–11.
44. Kamble PC, Sharma A, Singh V, Natraj B, Devani D, Khapane V. Outcome of single level disc prolapse treated with transforaminal steroid versus epidural steroid versus caudal steroids. Eur Spine J. 2016;25:217–21.
45. Ackerman WE 3rd, Ahmad M. The efficacy of lumbar epidural steroid injections in patients with lumbar disc herniations. Anesth Analg. 2007;104:1217–22.
46. Gharibo CG, Varlotta GP, Rhame EE, Liu EC, Bendo JA, Perloff MD. Interlaminar versus transforaminal epidural steroids for the treatment of subacute lumbar radicular pain: a randomized, blinded, prospective outcome study. Pain Physician. 2011;14:499–511.
47. Manchikanti L, Singh V, Pampati V, Falco FJ, Hirsch JA. Comparison of the efficacy of caudal, interlaminar, and transforaminal epidural injections in managing lumbar disc herniation: is one method superior to the other? Korean J Pain. 2015;28:11–21.
48. Vad VB, Bhat AL, Lutz GE, Cammisa F. Transforaminal epidural steroid injections in lumbosacral radiculopathy: a prospective randomized study. Spine (Phila Pa 1976). 2002;27:11–6.
49. Chang-Chien GC, Knezevic NN, McCormick Z, Chu SK, Trescot AM, Candido KD. Transforaminal versus interlaminar approaches to epidural steroid injections: a systematic review of comparative studies for lumbosacral radicular pain. Pain Physician. 2014;17:E509–24.
50. Ghai B, Vadaje KS, Wig J, Dhillon MS. Lateral parasagittal versus midline interlaminar lumbar epidural steroid injection for management of low back pain with lumbosacral radicular pain: a double-blind, randomized study. Anesth Analg. 2013;117:219–27.

51. Kim ED, Roh MS, Park JJ, Jo D. Comparison of the ventral epidural spreading in modified interlaminar approach and transforaminal approach: a randomized, double-blind study. Pain Med. 2016;17:1620–7.
52. Singh S, Kumar S, Chahal G, Verma R. Selective nerve root blocks vs. caudal epidural injection for single level prolapsed lumbar intervertebral disc - a prospective randomized study. J Clin Orthop Trauma. 2017;8:142–7.
53. Lee JH, Moon J, Lee SH. Comparison of effectiveness according to different approaches of epidural steroid injection in lumbosacral herniated disk and spinal stenosis. J Back Musculoskelet Rehabil. 2009;22:83–9.
54. Yoon JY, Kwon JW, Yoon YC, Lee J. Cervical interlaminar epidural steroid injection for unilateral cervical radiculopathy: comparison of midline and paramedian approaches for efficacy. Korean J Radiol. 2015;16:604–12.
55. Feeley IH, Healy EF, Noel J, Kiely PJ, Murphy TM. Particulate and non-particulate steroids in spinal epidurals: a systematic review and meta-analysis. Eur Spine J. 2017;26:336–44.
56. Mehta P, Syrop I, Singh JR, Kirschner J. Systematic review of the efficacy of particulate versus nonparticulate corticosteroids in epidural injections. PM R. 2017;9:502–12.

4 Medial Branch Block

Min Cheol Chang

4.1 Introduction

Facet (or zygapophyseal) joint-related pain is common in patients with a spinal disorder and occurs secondary to either facet joint wear and tear (degenerative change) or injury [1–4]. Pain secondary to facet joint pathology is not restricted to the facet joint; it can also spread to surrounding areas (i.e., referred pain) [5–7] (Fig. 4.1). Medial branch nerves are small nerves that feed out from the facet joints in the spine and transfer pain signals from the facet joints to the brain [8]. The medial branches of the dorsal rami innervate the facet joints, the posterior arches of the vertebrae, and certain spinal muscles (multifidus muscles) [9]. Of these, the facet joints are the only structure that can cause pain. Initially, a medial branch block was used to determine whether a patient's source of pain was of facet joint origin; however, several previous studies found that these blocks also reduce pain. Thus, MBNB are also used to alleviate facet joint-related pain.

The exact mechanism of the therapeutic effect of a medial branch block in reducing facet joint-related pain is unknown. However, suppression of the neural transmission of pain signals is known to be a key part of the mechanism. Local anesthetics, such as bupivacaine and lidocaine, and steroids are used as injection materials in medial branch blocks. Local anesthetics block axonal transport and suppress nociceptive discharge [10–14]. Steroids inhibit neural transmission within the nociceptive C-fibers [15–17].

M. C. Chang (✉)
Department of Physical Medicine and Rehabilitation, Yeungnam University Medical Center, Daegu, Republic of Korea

S.-H. Lee (ed.), *Minimally Invasive Spine Interventions*,
https://doi.org/10.1007/978-981-16-9547-6_4

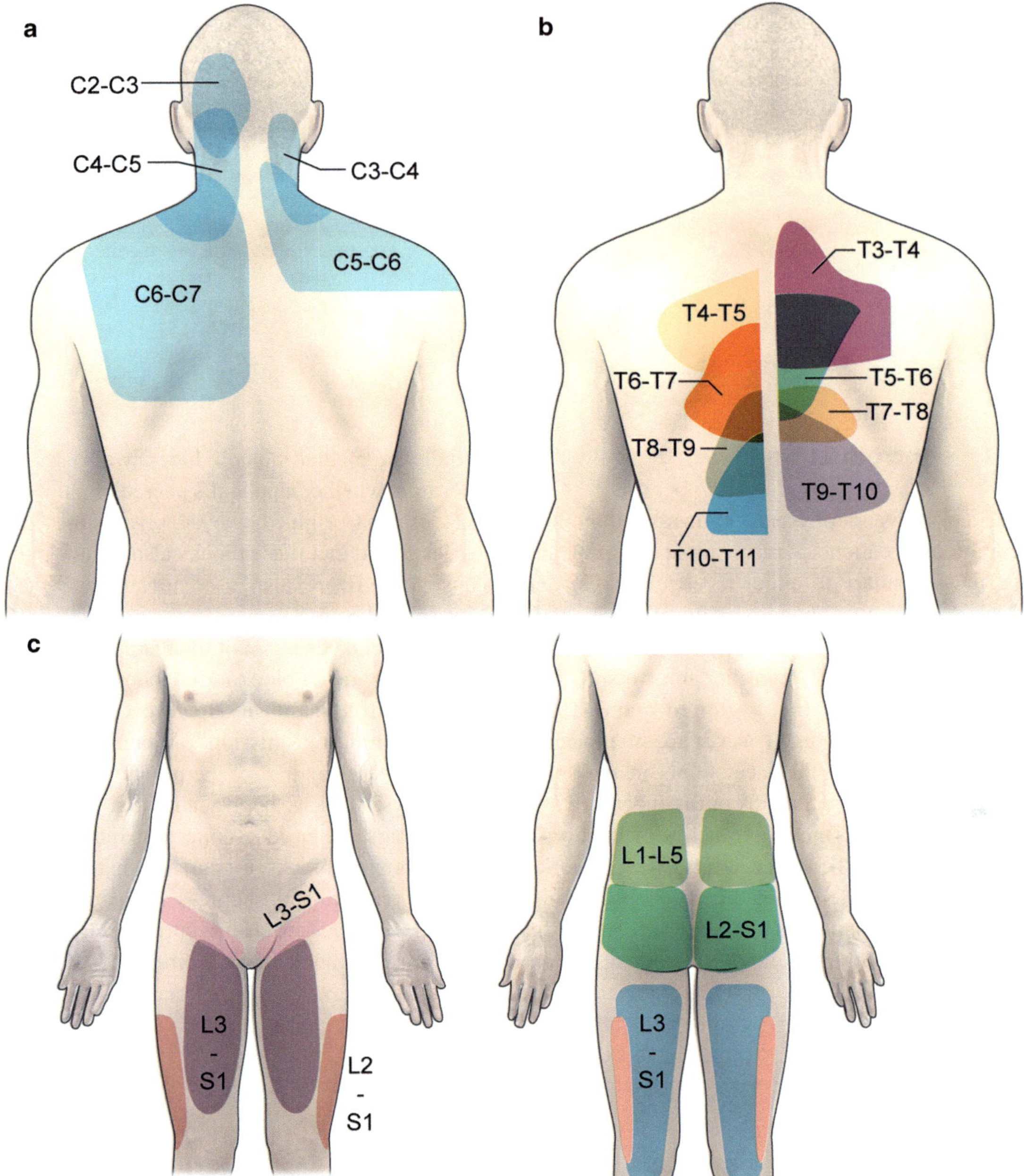

Fig. 4.1 Distribution of pain referred from the cervical, thoracic, and lumbar facet joints. C *cervical*, T *thoracic*, L *lumbar*, S *sacral*

4.2 Cervical Spine

4.2.1 Anatomical Considerations

Each cervical spinal dorsal ramus, except for the first, is divided into medial and lateral branches. The lateral branches supply the longissimus cervicis, splenius cervicis, and iliocostalis cervicis. Except for the first and second dorsal rami, the medial branch of each dorsal ramus passes posteriorly around an articular pillar and supplies the two adjacent facet joints and multifidus [18].

Accordingly, at typical cervical levels (C3–C4 to C6–C7 facet joints), each facet joint is innervated by articular branches from each of the two medial branches: one above and one below the joint [18]. For example, the C3 and C4 medial branches innervate the C3–C4 facet joint. Therefore, to block a facet joint within the range from C3–C4 to C6–C7, two medial branches should be blocked.

The medial branch of the third cervical spinal dorsal ramus divides into deep and superficial medial branches [19]. The deep medial branch curves dorsally and medially around the waist of the articular pillar and sends an articular branch to the C3–C4 facet joints. The superficial medial branch is the third occipital nerve, which curves around the lateral and dorsal surfaces of the C2–C3 facet joint and innervates it.

The course of the C7 medial branch varies, and it may appear at higher or lower locations of the C7 spine [20]. In the higher location, it passes the apex of the SAP of C7, and in the lower location, it passes the root of the C7 transverse process.

4.2.2 Techniques

A posterior approach is possible, but a lateral approach is simple and technically easy. The patient lies on his or her side with the painful area facing upward. A true lateral view of the cervical spine should be obtained (Fig. 4.2) with the fluoroscope aligned such that the target point is at the center of the X-ray beam. If the clinician does not have the correct lateral view, the needle may point to the opposite side. The needle entry point and surrounding area are sterilized. The clinician then blocks the two vertically adjacent spinal medial branches that innervate the target cervical facet joint.

4.2.2.1 C3–C6 Medial Branch Block (Fig. 4.2)

1. The target is the center of the articular pillar of the same segment as the target nerve. This point is where the two diagonals of the articular pillar meet.
2. The needle is inserted just above the target, and the C-arm fluoroscopy perspective is

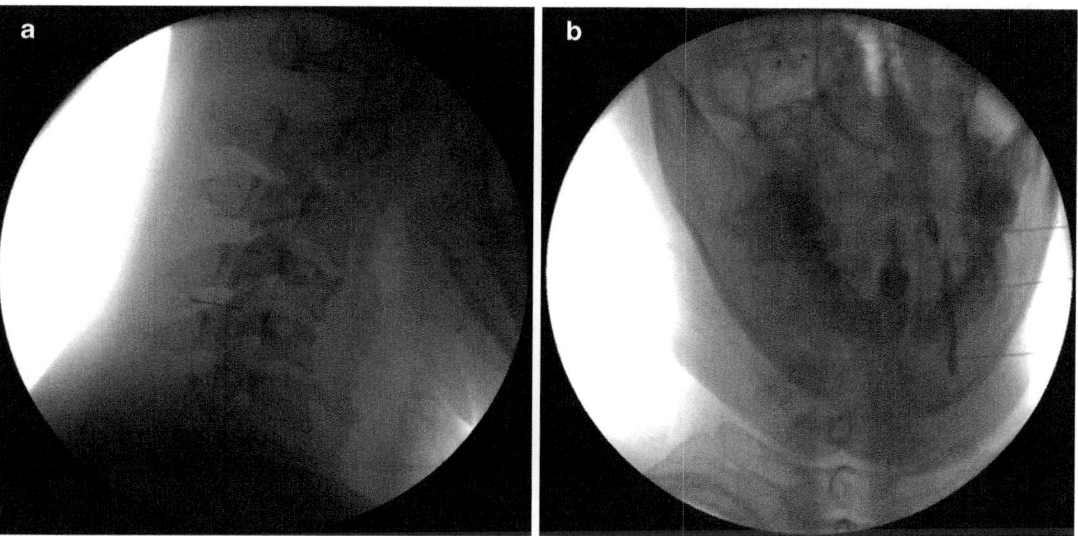

Fig. 4.2 Fluoroscopy-guided left C4–C6 cervical medial branch block: lateral view showing needles in each target (**a**) and anteroposterior view after the injection of contrast medium (**b**)

aligned to a straight line such that the needle appears close to the target. The needle is then slowly advanced until it reaches the articular pillar.
3. The needle tip location is confirmed by AP and lateral views on C-arm fluoroscopy. Contrast medium (0.2 mL) is injected to confirm that the needle is not inserted intravenously and that contrast medium is spreading across the side and filling the waist of the corresponding articular pillar.
4. In a diagnostic block performed to identify the painful cervical joint, lidocaine (0.5 mL) is injected into each medial branch. In a block sufficient for treatment, the local anesthetic is combined with a steroid, and the mixture (up to 2 mL) is injected into each medial branch.

4.2.2.2 C7 Medial Branch Block

1. A single target does not guarantee a successful C7 medial branch block because of this branch's anatomical variation; the nerve can cross the articular pillar at a high, low, or superficial level. Therefore, three target points are required for a C7 medial branch block (Fig. 4.3). One point lies at the base of the SAP, above the transverse process; the second lies on the apex of the SAP, and the third is collinear with and 3–5 mm superficial to the second.
2. The methods for needle insertion and contrast injection are the same as those for a C3–C6 medial branch block.
3. In a diagnostic block of the C7 medial branch, lidocaine (0.3 mL) is injected into each of the three target points.

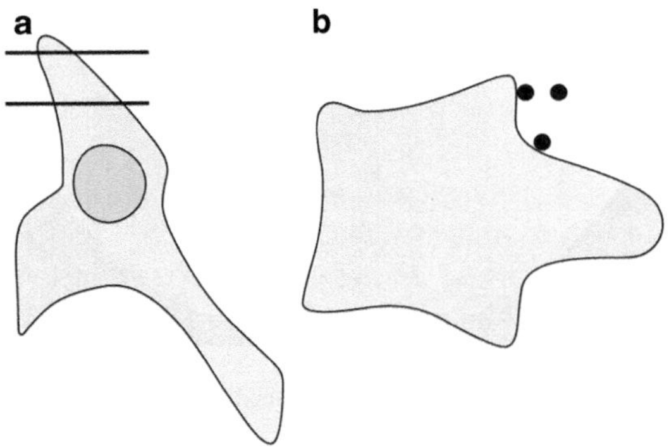

Fig. 4.3 Three possible locations (*black lines* and *dots*) of the C7 medial branch: lateral view of the C7 articular pillar and C7 transverse process (**a**) and anteroposterior view of the C7 articular pillar and transverse process (**b**)

4.2.3 Complications

Complications after a cervical medial branch block are rare, and there are few published reports of post-procedure complications. However, potential complications include an allergic reaction to the contrast solution or local anesthetic, hematoma, infection, and injection site discomfort. Cervical spinal cord injury has also been reported as a possible complication after a cervical medial branch block [21].

4.3 Thoracic Spine

4.3.1 Anatomical Considerations

At each thoracic segmental level, the thoracic dorsal rami pass dorsally and inferiorly through an aperture bound by the transverse processes superiorly and inferiorly, the facet joint medially, and the superior costotransverse ligament laterally. Thereafter, the thoracic dorsal rami divide into the medial and lateral branches [22]. The lateral branches pass laterally and supply several thoracic back muscles, including the levatores costarum, longissimus thoracis, iliocostalis, and spinalis. Each medial branch curves dorsally through the intertransverse space, crosses the superolateral corners of the transverse process, and then passes medially and inferiorly across the posterior surfaces of the transverse process [22]. After that, the nerve supplies the thoracic facet joints.

Each thoracic facet joint is innervated by the medial branch nerve of the same segment of the dorsal ramus and by the medial branch nerve that originates from the dorsal ramus of the upper thoracic spine [23]. Therefore, to fully control the pain caused by one facet joint, the two medial branch nerves must be blocked. For example, T4–T5 facet joint pain is managed by blocking the T3 and T4 medial branches.

4.3.2 Thoracic Medial Branch Block

1. The patient is placed prone on the fluoroscopy table.
2. The target thoracic vertebra is examined using the AP view on C-arm fluoroscopy, and the view is adjusted until the endplate of the disc on the target line is straight and the superolateral portion of the transverse process is visible.
3. After aseptic skin preparation, a 25-gauge needle is advanced until the target is reached. The targets (listed below) are based on the anatomical location (Figs. 4.4 and 4.5).
   - Branches T1–T4, T9, and T10: superolateral corners of the thoracic transverse processes.
   - Branches T5–T8: the rib (slightly above the superolateral ends of the transverse process) at the same depth as the back of the transverse process.
   - Branches T11 and T12: the junction of the superior articular and transverse processes.
4. The needle position is verified in the AP and lateral views, and an aspiration test is performed to confirm the absence of blood or spinal fluid leakage.
5. Contrast medium (0.1–1 mL) is injected to confirm the needle location.

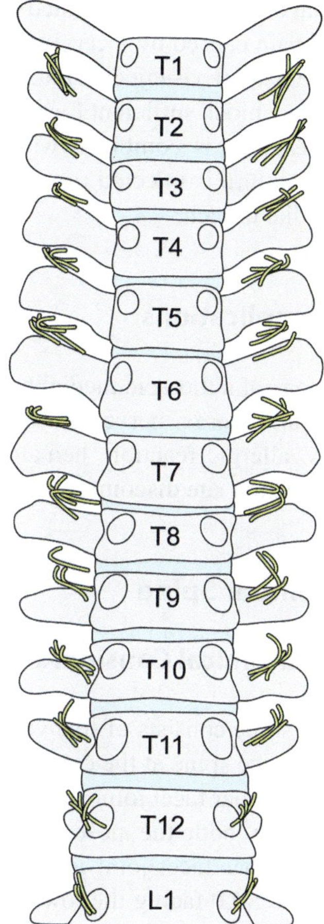

Fig. 4.4 The location of the thoracic medial branches

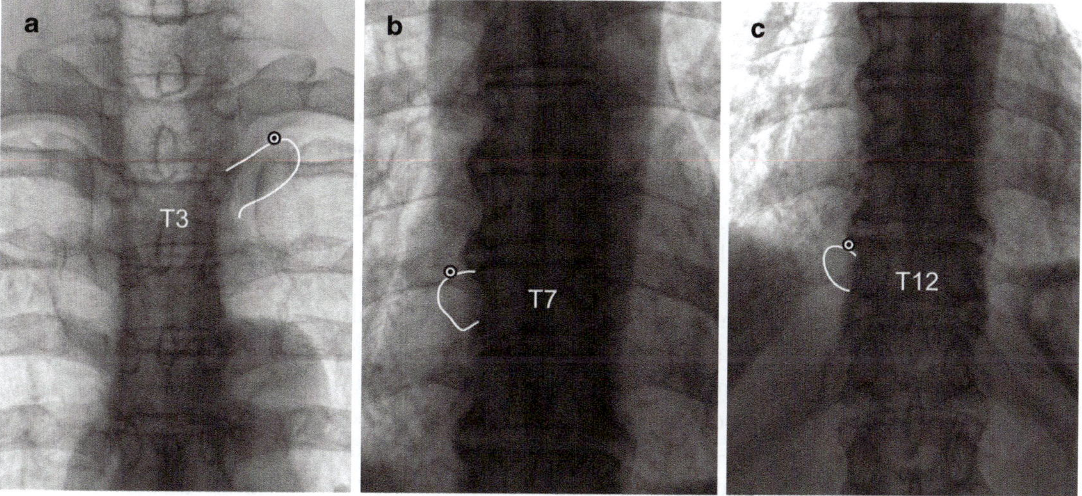

Fig. 4.5 Fluoroscopy-guided images showing thoracic medial branch block targets (*red dots*): upper thoracic, middle thoracic, and lower thoracic

6. For a diagnostic block performed to differentiate the pain caused by a cervical facet joint, lidocaine (0.5 mL) is injected into each medial branch. In a block sufficient for treatment, the local anesthetic is combined with a steroid, and the mixture is injected (up to 2 mL) into each medial branch.

4.3.3 Complications

Complications of a thoracic medial branch block include pneumothorax, nerve root injury, spinal cord injury, allergic reaction, hematoma, infection, and injection site discomfort.

4.4 Lumbar Spine

4.4.1 Anatomical Considerations

The lumbar spine consists of five vertebrae. The IVD supports the spine at the center in the front, whereas the lumbar facet joint supports the spine in the back on both the posterior and lateral sides. The lumbar facet joint is a true synovial joint, with the SAP facing the lower posteromedial lumbar spine and the inferior articular process facing the upper anterolateral lumbar spine [24]. The lumbar facet joint contains a synovial membrane and hyaline cartilage surfaces and is surrounded by a fibrous joint capsule. The volume of a lumbar facet joint is approximately 1–1.5 mL [25].

The L1 to L4 dorsal rami are short nerves that arise from the lumbar spinal nerves (Fig. 4.6). Each nerve runs back toward the upper border of the subjacent transverse process. The L5 dorsal ramus is longer and passes over the top of the ala of the sacrum [8, 26]. The L1–L4 dorsal rami divide into medial, intermediate, and lateral branches as they travel across their transverse processes [26]. The L5 dorsal ramus divides into a medial branch and a branch equivalent to the intermediate branches of the L1–L4 dorsal rami. The lateral and intermediate branches innervate the iliocostalis lumborum and longissimus muscles. The medial branches of the lumbar dorsal rami innervate the lumbar facet joints. These pass across the top of their respective transverse processes. Each nerve runs along the bone at the junction of the base of the transverse process and root of the SAP [26]. Subsequently, each medial branch curves medially around the base of the SAP and finally crosses the vertebral lamina to divide into multiple branches that innervate the multifidus muscle, interspinous muscle, and paraspinal ligaments as well as the two facet joints above and below its course [25].

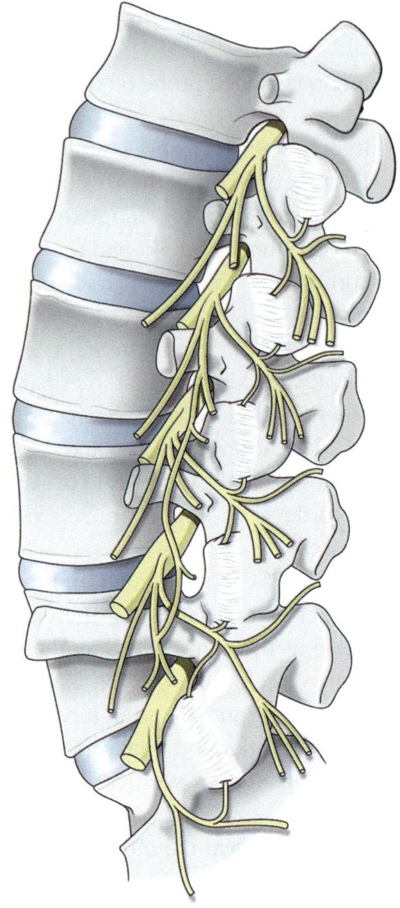

Fig. 4.6 Left posterior view of the lumbar spine showing branches of the lumbar dorsal rami. *DR*, dorsal ramus; *ib*, intermediate branch; *ibp*, intermediate branch plexus; *lb*, lateral branch; *mb*, medial branch; *a*, articular branch; *VR*, ventral ramus

The L5 medial branch crosses the ala of the sacrum and passes along the groove formed by the junction of the sacral ala and root of the SAP of the sacrum [26]. After that, the nerve curves medially around the base of the L5–S1 facet joint and supplies an articular branch to this joint. Two medial branches must be blocked to block each lumbar facet joint. For example, the L4–L5 facet joint treatment requires targeting the junction of the superior articular and transverse processes of L4 and L5 (i.e., L3 and L4 medial branches). The L5–S1 facet joint treatment is accomplished by conducting the block at the transverse process of L5 and the junction of the ala of the sacrum and the SAP of S1 (i.e., the L4 and L5 medial branches).

4.4.2 Lumbar Medial Branch Block (Fig. 4.7)

1. The patient is placed prone on the fluoroscopy table.
2. The target area of the lumbar spine is evaluated in the AP view on C-arm fluoroscopy. The view is adjusted until the endplate of the disc above the target point appears straight, and the C-arm is then turned 25°–30° in the direction of the target facet joint such that the

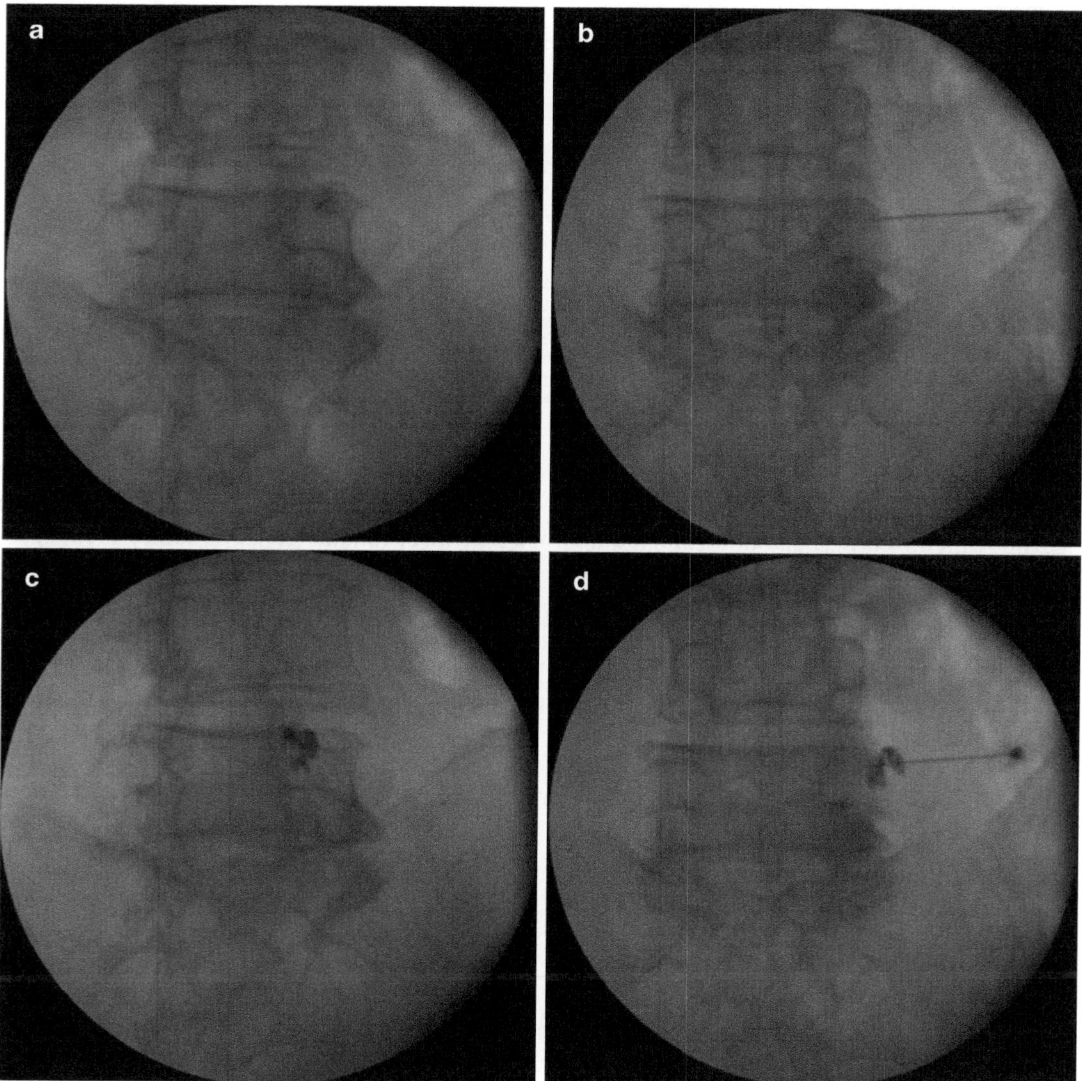

Fig. 4.7 Fluoroscopy-guided right lumbar vertebra 4 medial branch block: the oblique (**a**) and anteroposterior (**b**) views show the needle inserted in the target, and the oblique (**c**) and anteroposterior (**d**) views show the results of contrast medium injection

articular surface of the lumbar facet is clearly visible.

3. In an L1–L4 medial branch block, the needle tip is directed towards the junction of the SAP and the transverse process and advanced until it reaches the bone. A "Scottie dog" image is visible, with the target point lying at the "eye" of the "dog." In an L5 medial branch block, the needle tip should reach the junction of the sacral ala and the root of the SAP of the sacrum.
4. A contrast agent (0.5 mL) is injected, and the operator confirms the absence of intravascular spread. During a lumbar medial branch block, the incidence of intravascular uptake is approximately 6% per nerve.
5. In a diagnostic block, lidocaine (0.5 mL) is injected into each medial branch. In a therapeutic block, the local anesthetic is combined with a steroid, and the mixture is injected (up to 2 mL) into each medial branch.

4.4.3 Complications

A lumbar medial branch block is a relatively safe procedure. There are no structures that can be injured during the passage of the needle. However, potential complications include an allergic reaction to the contrast solution or local anesthetics, hematoma, infection, and injection site discomfort.

4.5 Discussion

4.5.1 Cervical Medial Branch Block

Neck pain of cervical facet joint origin is most frequently diagnosed using a cervical medial branch block. A cervical medial branch block is typically considered diagnostic if the patient experiences pain reduction of 80% for at least 2 h after lidocaine injection and 3 h after bupivacaine administration, although some studies suggest that 50% pain reduction is a useful criterion for the diagnosis of neck pain of cervical facet joint origin. Most previous studies have used 0.5 mL of local anesthetic for diagnostic medial branch blocks. However, in 2010, Cohen et al. showed that using an injection volume of 0.25 mL of local anesthetic instead of 0.5 mL can improve diagnostic precision and accuracy [20]. They found that when performing a block using 0.5 mL of local anesthetic, the medication extended to other structures and caused neck pain in several cases. Thus, the authors recommended reducing the injection volume for diagnostic cervical medial branch blocks.

Manchikanti et al. performed three RCTs of therapeutic cervical medial branch blocks from 2006 to 2010 and reported that a therapeutic medial branch block was effective in treating chronic cervical facet joint pain [27–29]. In their studies, blocks using bupivacaine both with and without a steroid effectively controlled chronic neck pain of facet joint origin. The pain-reducing effects of therapeutic local anesthetic medial branch blocks with and without steroids were not significantly different. Manchikanti et al. also showed that the effect of a therapeutic medial branch block could last for one to 2 years after injection. In 2010, Klessinger conducted a therapeutic medial branch block (local anesthetic and steroid) in 312 patients with persistent neck pain after cervical spinal surgery and followed them for at least 6 months [30]. The author's retrospective analysis of procedure outcomes showed that 52.9% of patients were successfully treated. In 2016, Persson et al. prospectively evaluated the effect of a cervical medial branch block using 0.5 mL of bupivacaine in 47 patients with chronic neck pain due to a whiplash injury [31]. After injection, only approximately 30% of patients showed a positive response.

Although the evidence may be insufficient, positive outcomes after therapeutic cervical medial branch blocks in several previous studies indicate that the procedure could be a good option for alleviating cervical facet joint pain [27–31]. Additional well-designed RCTs should be conducted to clarify the therapeutic effectiveness of a cervical medial branch block for cervical facet joint pain and determine appropriate criteria for the procedure. Moreover, some studies have reported that blocks using a combination of local anesthetic and a steroid show therapeutic effects similar to blocks with local anesthetic alone; however, further studies are necessary to clarify this issue.

Medial branch blocks are increasingly performed under ultrasound guidance [32]. Ultrasound-guided injections have the merits of eliminating the risk of radiation exposure and decreased procedure time.

4.5.2 Thoracic Medial Branch Block

There are fewer studies of thoracic medial branch blocks than of cervical and lumbar medial branch blocks because the incidence of thoracic facet joint pain is relatively lower than that of cervical or lumbar facet joint pain. Previous studies found that patients with temporary pain reduction ≥80% after a diagnostic thoracic medial branch block with local anesthetic have thoracic facet joint pain. Manchikanti et al. performed four prospective studies to evaluate therapeutic thoracic medial branch blocks [33–36]. In 2006, they conducted therapeutic thoracic medial branch blocks using bupivacaine mixed with a steroid (total 1–1.5 mL mixture) in 55 patients with chronic thoracic facet joint pain. After the procedure, about 70% of patients experienced ≥50% pain relief [33]. In 2008, the same authors recruited 48 patients with thoracic facet joint pain and divided them into groups receiving a local anesthetic (bupivacaine) or local anesthetic and a steroid (bupivacaine and betamethasone). In both groups, approximately 80% of patients reported ≥50% pain relief 1 year after their procedure [34]. In 2010, Manchikanti et al. found functional improvement (measured with the Oswestry Disability Index) in addition to pain reduction in 90% of 100 study patients 1 year after a therapeutic medial branch block using bupivacaine with or without betamethasone (total 0.5–1 mL mixture) [35]. In 2012, the authors observed long-term pain reduction and functional improvement after thoracic medial branch blocks performed 2 years earlier [36]. Interestingly, in 2018, Lee et al. compared therapeutic medial branch blocks with intra-articular thoracic facet joint injections in 20 patients divided into two subgroups [23]. Both groups showed significant pain relief one, three, and 6 months after each treatment, and the effects of the two procedures were similar.

Taken together, the findings of these previous studies indicate that the therapeutic thoracic medial branch block seems to be a beneficial treatment option for thoracic facet joint pain. However, most studies have included a limited sample size. Therefore, further research should be conducted to confirm the effectiveness of thoracic medial branch blocks.

4.5.3 Lumbar Medial Branch Block

Research has demonstrated the positive diagnostic value of a lumbar medial branch block for lumbar facet joint-related back pain. In 1998, Kaplan et al. showed that a lumbar medial branch block had high diagnostic accuracy (over 90%) for lumbar facet joint-related neck pain [37]. In 2007, Birkenmaier et al. demonstrated that a lumbar medial branch block is superior to a pericapsular block for the diagnosis of lumbar facet joint pain [38].

Manchikanti et al. performed several prospective studies of therapeutic lumbar medial branch blocks [39–41]. They recruited patients with ≥80% pain relief after a diagnostic lumbar medial branch block with local anesthetic (0.5 mL) and conducted therapeutic medial branch blocks. In all studies, the authors found that therapeutic lumbar medial branch blocks using bupivacaine with or without a steroid (total 0.5–1 mL) effectively controlled chronic lumbar facet joint pain; studies by other authors confirmed this positive pain-reducing effect [32, 42].

Recently, as more physicians have gained experience with musculoskeletal ultrasound, the use of ultrasound-guided lumbar medial branch blocks has become widespread, and this treatment has the same pain-reducing effect as a fluoroscopy-guided medial branch block [42, 43]. Further prospective clinical trials are necessary to evaluate the wider application of lumbar medial branch blocks for the treatment of lumbar facet joint pain.

References

1. Manchikanti L, Pampati V, Fellows B, Baha AG. The inability of the clinical picture to characterize pain from facet joints. Pain Physician. 2000;3:158–66.
2. Manchikanti L, Pampati V, Fellows B, Bakhit CE. Prevalence of lumbar facet joint pain in chronic low back pain. Pain Physician. 1999;2:59–64.
3. Schwarzer AC, Aprill CN, Derby R, Fortin J, Kine G, Bogduk N. Clinical features of patients with pain stemming from the lumbar zygapophyseal joints. Is the lumbar facet syndrome a clinical entity? Spine (Phila Pa 1976). 1994;19:1132–7.
4. Jaumard NV, Welch WC, Winkelstein BA. Spinal facet joint biomechanics and mechanotransduction in normal, injury and degenerative conditions. J Biomech Eng. 2011;133:071010.
5. Dreyfuss P, Tibiletti C, Dreyer SJ. Thoracic zygapophyseal joint pain patterns. A study in normal volunteers. Spine (Phila Pa 1976). 1994;19:807–11.
6. Lim JW, Cho YW, Lee DG, Chang MC. Comparison of intraarticular pulsed radiofrequency and intraarticular corticosteroid injection for management of cervical facet joint pain. Pain Physician. 2017;20:E961–7.
7. Perolat R, Kastler A, Nicot B, Pellat JM, Tahon F, Attye A, et al. Facet joint syndrome: from diagnosis to interventional management. Insights Imaging. 2018;9:773–89.
8. Shuang F, Hou SX, Zhu JL, Liu Y, Zhou Y, Zhang CL, et al. Clinical anatomy and measurement of the medial branch of the spinal dorsal ramus. Medicine (Baltimore). 2015;94:e2367.
9. Sihvonen T, Lindgren KA, Airaksinen O, Leino E, Partanen J, Hänninen O. Dorsal ramus irritation associated with recurrent low back pain and its relief with local anesthetic or training therapy. J Spinal Disord. 1995;8:8–14.
10. Arnér S, Lindblom U, Meyerson BA, Molander C. Prolonged relief of neuralgia after regional anesthetic blocks. A call for further experimental and systematic clinical studies. Pain. 1990;43:287–97.
11. Bisby MA. Inhibition of axonal transport in nerves chronically treated with local anesthetics. Exp Neurol. 1975;47:481–9.
12. Katz WA, Rothenberg R. Section 3: the nature of pain: pathophysiology. J Clin Rheumatol. 2005;11(2 Suppl):S11–5.
13. Lavoie PA, Khazen T, Filion PR. Mechanisms of the inhibition of fast axonal transport by local anesthetics. Neuropharmacology. 1989;28:175–81.
14. Melzack R, Coderre TJ, Katz J, Vaccarino AL. Central neuroplasticity and pathological pain. Ann N Y Acad Sci. 2001;933:157–74.
15. Hayashi N, Weinstein JN, Meller ST, Lee HM, Spratt KF, Gebhart GF. The effect of epidural injection of betamethasone or bupivacaine in a rat model of lumbar radiculopathy. Spine (Phila Pa 1976). 1998;23:877–85.
16. Lee HM, Weinstein JN, Meller ST, Hayashi N, Spratt KF, Gebhart GF. The role of steroids and their effects on phospholipase A2. An animal model of radiculopathy. Spine (Phila Pa 1976). 1998;23:1191–6.
17. Pasqualucci A, Varrassi G, Braschi A, Peduto VA, Brunelli A, Marinangeli F, et al. Epidural local anesthetic plus corticosteroid for the treatment of cervical brachial radicular pain: single injection versus continuous infusion. Clin J Pain. 2007;23:551–7.
18. Ebraheim NA, Haman ST, Xu R, Yeasting RA. The anatomic location of the dorsal ramus of the cervical nerve and its relation to the superior articular process of the lateral mass. Spine (Phila Pa 1976). 1998;23:1968–71.
19. Narouze SN, Provenzano DA. Sonographically guided cervical facet nerve and joint injections: why sonography? J Ultrasound Med. 2013;32:1885–96.
20. Cohen SP, Strassels SA, Kurihara C, Forsythe A, Buckenmaier CC 3rd, McLean B, et al. Randomized study assessing the accuracy of cervical facet joint nerve (medial branch) blocks using different injectate volumes. Anesthesiology. 2010;112:144–52.
21. Park D, Seong MY, Kim HY, Ryu JS. Spinal cord injury during ultrasound-guided C7 cervical medial branch block. Am J Phys Med Rehabil. 2017;96:e111–4.
22. Chua WH, Bogduk N. The surgical anatomy of thoracic facet denervation. Acta Neurochir. 1995;136:140–4.
23. Lee DG, Ahn SH, Cho YW, Do KH, Kwak SG, Chang MC. Comparison of intra-articular thoracic facet joint steroid injection and thoracic medial branch block for the management of thoracic facet joint pain. Spine (Phila Pa 1976). 2018;43:76–80.
24. Gellhorn AC, Katz JN, Suri P. Osteoarthritis of the spine: the facet joints. Nat Rev Rheumatol. 2013;9:216–24.
25. Cohen SP, Raja SN. Pathogenesis, diagnosis, and treatment of lumbar zygapophyseal (facet) joint pain. Anesthesiology. 2007;106:591–614.
26. Saito T, Steinke H, Miyaki T, Nawa S, Umemoto K, Miyakawa K, et al. Analysis of the posterior ramus of the lumbar spinal nerve: the structure of the posterior ramus of the spinal nerve. Anesthesiology. 2013;118:88–94.
27. Manchikanti L, Damron K, Cash K, Manchukonda R, Pampati V. Therapeutic cervical medial branch blocks in managing chronic neck pain: a preliminary report of a randomized, double-blind, controlled trial: clinical trial NCT0033272. Pain Physician. 2006;9:333–46.
28. Manchikanti L, Singh V, Falco FJ, Cash KM, Fellows B. Cervical medial branch blocks for chronic cervical facet joint pain: a randomized, double-blind, controlled trial with one-year follow-up. Spine (Phila Pa 1976). 2008;33:1813–20.
29. Manchikanti L, Singh V, Falco FJ, Cash KA, Fellows B. Comparative outcomes of a 2-year follow-up of cervical medial branch blocks in management of chronic neck pain: a randomized, double-blind controlled trial. Pain Physician. 2010;13:437–50.

30. Klessinger S. The benefit of therapeutic medial branch blocks after cervical operations. Pain Physician. 2010;13:527–34.
31. Persson M, Sörensen J, Gerdle B. Chronic whiplash associated disorders (WAD): responses to nerve blocks of cervical zygapophyseal joints. Pain Med. 2016;17:2162–75.
32. Park KD, Lim DJ, Lee WY, Ahn J, Park Y. Ultrasound versus fluoroscopy-guided cervical medial branch block for the treatment of chronic cervical facet joint pain: a retrospective comparative study. Skelet Radiol. 2017;46:81–91.
33. Manchikanti L, Manchikanti KN, Manchukonda R, Pampati V, Cash KA. Evaluation of therapeutic thoracic medial branch block effectiveness in chronic thoracic pain: a prospective outcome study with minimum 1-year follow up. Pain Physician. 2006;9:97–105.
34. Manchikanti L, Singh V, Falco FJ, Cash KA, Pampati V. Effectiveness of thoracic medial branch blocks in managing chronic pain: a preliminary report of a randomized, double-blind controlled trial. Pain Physician. 2008;11:491–504.
35. Manchikanti L, Singh V, Falco FJ, Cash KA, Pampati V, Fellows B. Comparative effectiveness of a one-year follow-up of thoracic medial branch blocks in management of chronic thoracic pain: a randomized, double-blind active controlled trial. Pain Physician. 2010;13:535–48.
36. Manchikanti L, Singh V, Falco FJ, Cash KA, Pampati V, Fellows B. The role of thoracic medial branch blocks in managing chronic mid and upper back pain: a randomized, double-blind, active-control trial with a 2-year follow-up. Anesthesiol Res Pract. 2012;2012:585806.
37. Kaplan M, Dreyfuss P, Halbrook B, Bogduk N. The ability of lumbar medial branch blocks to anesthetize the zygapophyseal joint. A physiologic challenge. Spine (Phila Pa 1976). 1998;23:1847–52.
38. Birkenmaier C, Veihelmann A, Trouillier HH, Hausdorf J, von Schulze PC. Medial branch blocks versus pericapsular blocks in selecting patients for percutaneous cryodenervation of lumbar facet joints. Reg Anesth Pain Med. 2007;32:27–33.
39. Manchikanti L, Singh V, Falco FJ, Cash KA, Pampati V. Evaluation of lumbar facet joint nerve blocks in managing chronic low back pain: a randomized, double-blind, controlled trial with a 2-year follow-up. Int J Med Sci. 2010;7:124–35.
40. Manchikanti L, Singh V, Falco FJ, Cash KA, Pampati V. Lumbar facet joint nerve blocks in managing chronic facet joint pain: one-year follow-up of a randomized, double-blind controlled trial: clinical trial NCT00355914. Pain Physician. 2008;11:121–32.
41. Manchikanti L, Manchikanti KN, Manchukonda R, Cash KA, Damron KS, Pampati V, et al. Evaluation of lumbar facet joint nerve blocks in the management of chronic low back pain: preliminary report of a randomized, double-blind controlled trial: clinical trial NCT00355914. Pain Physician. 2007;10:425–40.
42. Koh WU, Kim SH, Hwang BY, Choi WJ, Song JG, Suh JH, et al. Value of bone scintigraphy and single photon emission computed tomography (SPECT) in lumbar facet disease and prediction of short-term outcome of ultrasound guided medial branch block with bone SPECT. Korean J Pain. 2011;24:81–6.
43. Han SH, Park KD, Cho KR, Park Y. Ultrasound versus fluoroscopy-guided medial branch block for the treatment of lower lumbar facet joint pain: a retrospective comparative study. Medicine (Baltimore). 2017;96:e6655.

5 Intra-articular Injection: Z-Joint, Intradiscal, and Sacroiliac Joint

Yun-Woo Cho

5.1 Introduction

Intervertebral discs (IVDs), facet joints, and sacroiliac (SI) joints are connected and can be a source of axial spine pain with or without referred pain. Facet joints may also cause chronic lower back, posterior neck, and upper and middle back pain because they have free and encapsulated nerve endings, nerves containing pain-related peptides, and capsules containing low-threshold mechanoreceptors and mechanically sensitive nociceptors. Further, joint loading can substantially strain the joint capsule [1]. Compared with the lumbar spine facet joints, those in the cervical spine play a greater role in load-bearing, and the prevalence of discogenic pain in the cervical spine is only 16%, whereas the prevalence of cervical facet joint pain is approximately 65% [2].

The SI joint is a vertically oriented diarthrodial joint that may be susceptible to damage after unusual stress and strain. SI joint pain may result from inflammatory mediators of the joint and interosseous ligaments, and repetitive damage may sensitize the joint's abundant sensory innervation. In these cases, an SI joint steroid and local anesthetic injection can provide short-term pain relief [3].

Y.-W. Cho (✉)
Ahn, Sang-Ho Rehabilitation Clinic, Daegu, Republic of Korea

IVDs can also be a cause of low back pain (LBP) and neck pain. Discogenic LBP may be associated with the upregulation of proinflammatory cytokines and chemokines such as tumor necrosis factor-α, interleukin-1, interleukin-6, and others and sensory nerve ingrowth into the inner layer of the degenerated IVDs [4]. Intradiscal procedures such as intradiscal injection with steroid or biological agents are used to manage discogenic pain.

5.2 Cervical Spine

5.2.1 Anatomical Considerations

Cervical IVDs, cervical facet joints, and the atlanto-axial and atlanto-occipital joints may all contribute to posterior neck pain, upper extremity pain, and headaches.

The atlanto-occipital joint connects the convex occipital condyles and concave superior articular surfaces of the lateral mass of the atlas (C1) and has a medially concave c-shape. The lateral atlanto-axial joints are oriented in the axial plane and consist of the two convex articular processes of C1 and the axis (C2). The vertebral artery and the C2 ganglia lie very close to the atlanto-occipital and atlanto-axial joints. The vertebral arteries usually pass superiorly within the transverse foramen, from C6 or C7 toward C1, and then proceed superomedially to

S.-H. Lee (ed.), *Minimally Invasive Spine Interventions*,
https://doi.org/10.1007/978-981-16-9547-6_5

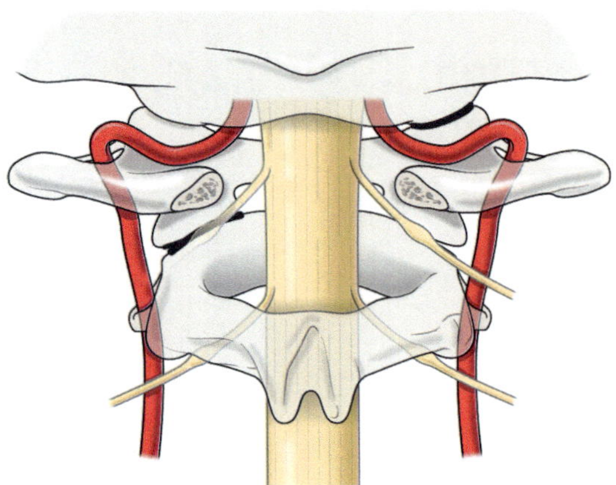

Fig. 5.1 The relationship of the vertebral artery to the atlanto-occipital and atlanto-axial joints: the vertebral arteries are located laterally at the atlanto-axial joint level and medially at the atlanto-occipital joint level

the foramen magnum. Consequently, the vertebral arteries are located laterally at the atlanto-axial joint level and medially at the atlanto-occipital joint level (Fig. 5.1) [5]. The C2 ganglion is confined within a foramen between the arch of the atlas and the lamina of the axis and lies within the needle trajectory for an atlanto-axial joint injection [6]. Cervical facet joints are oriented to the coronal plane. The angle from the coronal plane of the C2–C3 through C5–C6 facet joints is 35°, and that of the C6–C7 facet joint is 22° (Fig. 5.2) [7, 8].

The cervical disc is composed of periosteofascial tissue, fibers of the annulus fibrosus (AF), and a deep core of fibrocartilaginous material [9]. Because the esophagus is located slightly to the left immediately in front of the vertebral body and the carotid artery is near the cervical spine, intradiscal procedures are typically approached from the right side.

5.2.2 Techniques

5.2.2.1 Atlanto-Occipital Joint Injections

1. The patient lies prone with a pillow under the chest with neck flexion as close as possible to 30° from the table.
2. The C-arm is rotated ipsilaterally and tilted cranially from the sagittal and axial planes, about 30° respectively. A 25-gauge, 3.5-inch spinal needle is inserted into the lateral third of the occipital condyle of the atlanto-occipital joint while carefully avoiding the vertebral artery.
3. After the needle contacts the bone, the C-arm is rotated approximately 30° contralaterally.
4. The needle is withdrawn slightly and then advanced to the joint cavity.
5. When the needle tip is within the atlanto-occipital joint, contrast (approximately 0.5 cc) is injected and needle placement confirmed by a bright ellipsoid of contrast in the contralateral view on an arthrogram (Fig. 5.3).
6. A mixture of local anesthetic and a steroid (approximately 1 mL) is carefully injected.

5.2.2.2 Lateral Atlanto-Axial Joint Injections

1. The patient lies prone with a pillow under the forehead.
2. The C-arm is tilted slightly in the cranial or caudal direction until the joint margin is identified (with the patient's mouth open if the joint is obscured by teeth) (Fig. 5.4a).
3. A 25-gauge, 3.5-inch spinal needle is inserted and advanced toward the lateral third of the SAP of the joint while avoiding the medially located C2 ganglia, spinal cord, and laterally located vertebral artery (Fig. 5.4b).
4. The needle depth is monitored by rotating the C-arm laterally, and the needle is advanced until the tip reaches the joint (Fig. 5.4c).
5. Contrast is injected, and the needle position is confirmed by the presence of a circle of contrast and a linear contrast pattern on the lateral and AP arthrograms, respectively (Fig. 5.4d, e).
6. A mixture of local anesthetic and a steroid (approximately 1 mL) is carefully injected.

5.2.2.3 C2-C3–C6-C7 Facet Joint Injection

1. The patient lies prone with the neck rotated to expose the target facet joint from chin (if the

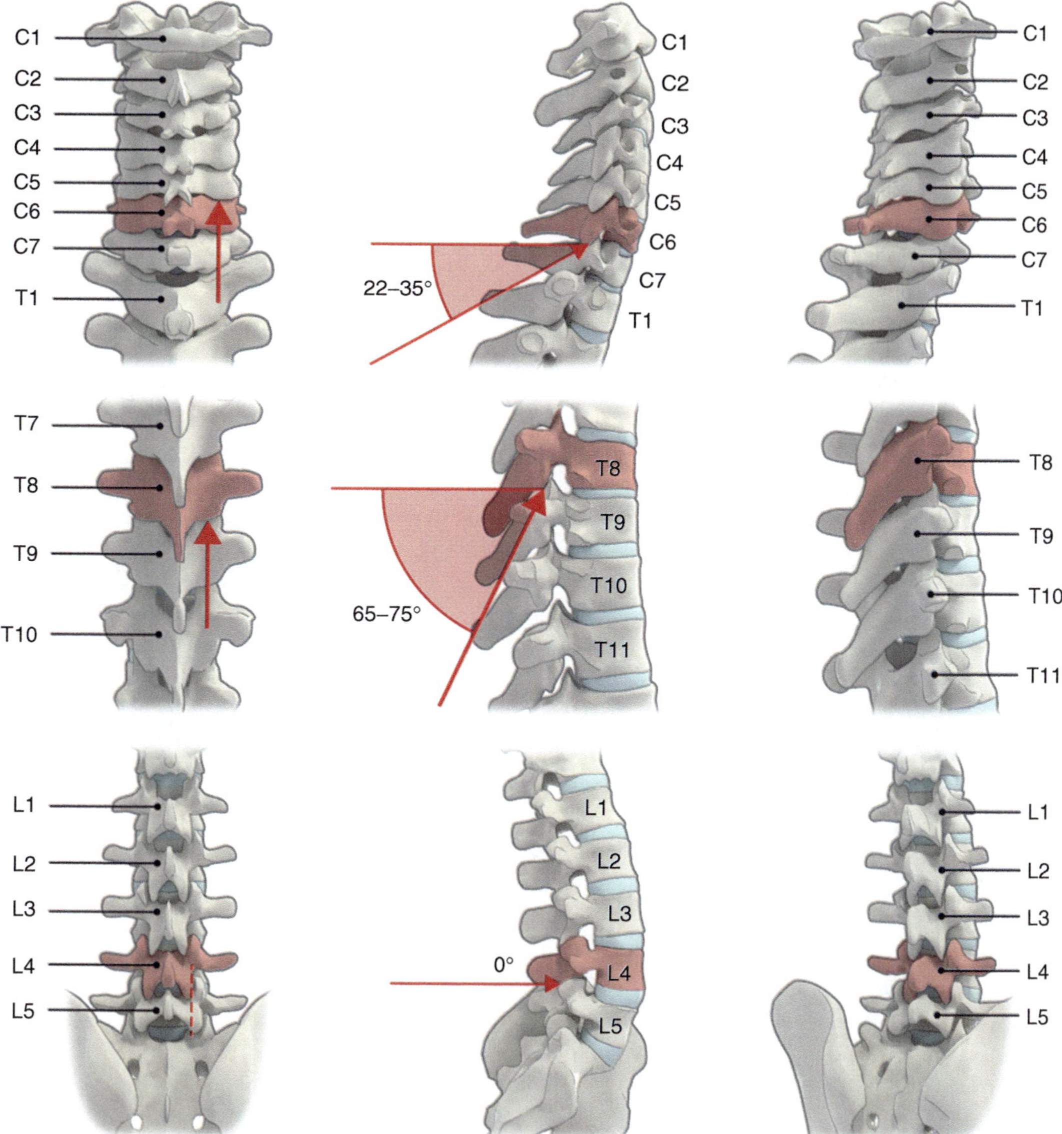

Fig. 5.2 Cervical, thoracic, and lumbosacral facet joint orientation and needle approach angles for facet joint injections: cervical facet joints are oriented to the coronal plane, and the angle of each cervical facet joint is 22° to 35° from the coronal plane, respectively; thoracic facet joints are nearly vertical and coronal in orientation, rotating towards the sagittal plane near the thoracolumbar junction; at T11–T12 and the thoracolumbar junction, the orientation becomes slightly more sagittal, and each facet joint is angled between 65° and 75° from the transverse plane

target is the left C5–6 facet joint, the neck is rotated to the right side).

2. The C-arm is tilted caudally approximately 30°.
3. A 25-gauge, 3.5-inch spinal needle is advanced toward the target joint.
4. The C-arm is rotated laterally after the needle contacts the bone.
5. The needle is withdrawn slightly and then advanced to the joint cavity.
6. After the needle enters the target joint, contrast is injected, and the tip position is confirmed

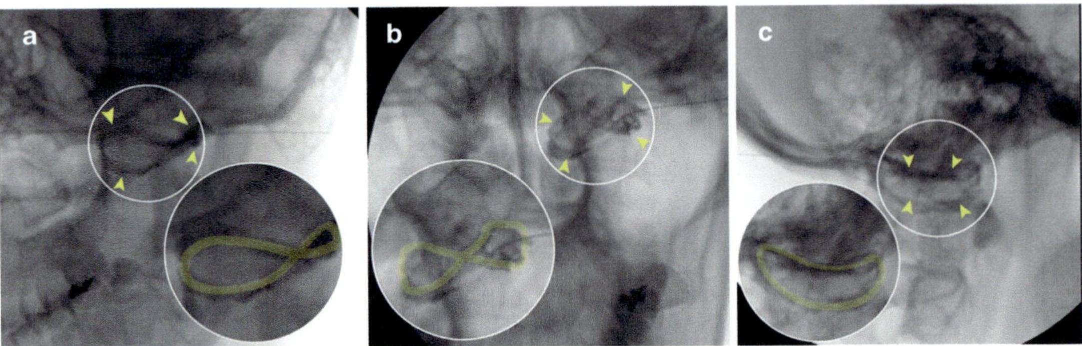

Fig. 5.3 C-arm guided atlanto-occipital joint injection: an ellipsoid of contrast is seen on arthrograms in contralateral (**a**), anteroposterior (**b**), and lateral views (**c**)

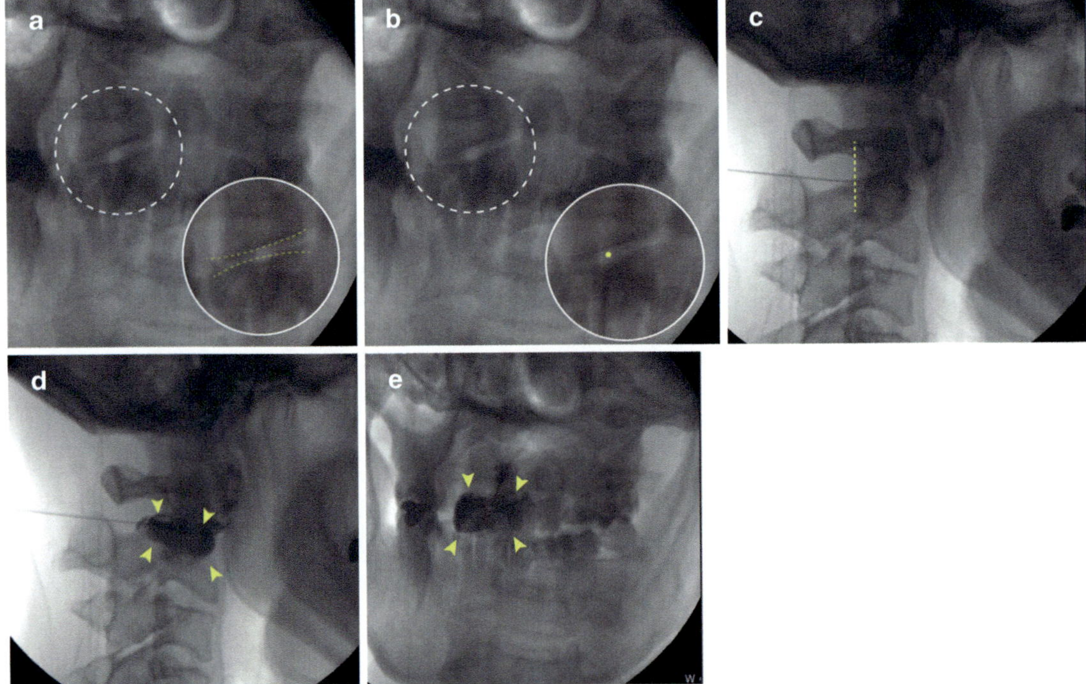

Fig. 5.4 C-arm-guided lateral atlanto-axial joint injection (see above)

by a linear contrast pattern in the lateral view on an arthrogram (Fig. 5.5).

7. A mixture of local anesthetic and a steroid (approximately 1 mL) is carefully injected.

5.2.2.4 Intradiscal Injection

1. The patient lies supine with slight extension and contralateral rotation of the neck.
2. The C-arm is placed in the AP position and tilted to identify the upper and lower end-plates of the target IVD.
3. The esophagus and trachea are identified medial to the internal carotid artery, and then the needle entry point is selected between these structures and the internal carotid artery (typically, a right-side anterolateral approach is preferred).

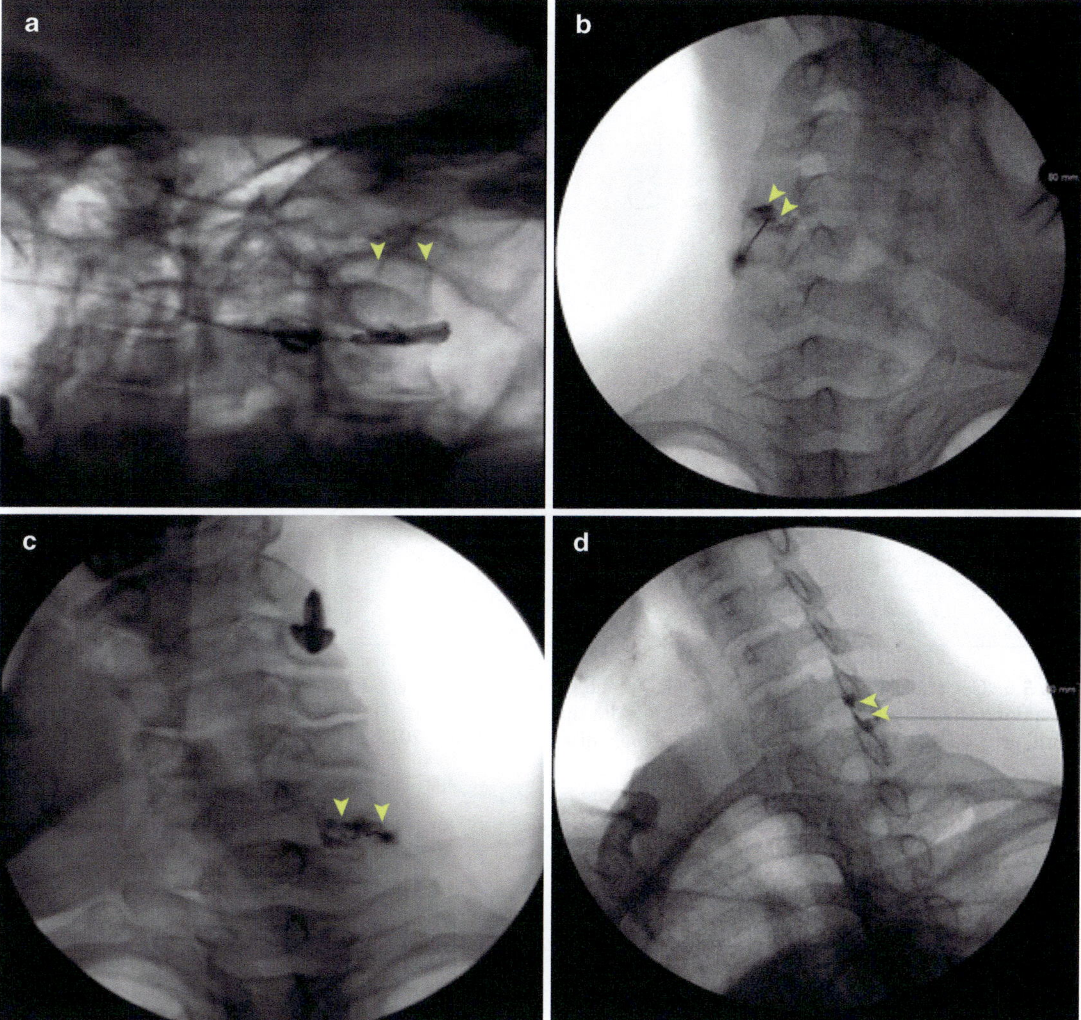

Fig. 5.5 Cervical facet joint arthrograms: right C2–C3 facet (**a**), left C4–C5 facet (**b**), and right C6–C7 facet joints (**c**) in the anteroposterior view and the C7–T1 facet joint in the lateral view (**d**) C, cervical

4. With AP and lateral C-arm guidance, a 25-gauge, 3.5-inch spinal needle is carefully advanced toward the upper endplate of the target disc until the tip contacts the bone.
5. The needle is withdrawn slightly and then moved to the center of the IVD again, with AP and lateral C-arm guidance.
6. Contrast (approximately 0.5 mL) is injected, and a discogram is obtained to confirm the needle tip position (Fig. 5.6).
7. A mixture of local anesthetic and a steroid (approximately 1 mL) is carefully injected [10].

5.2.3 Complications

Complications after facet joint injections are uncommon. However, infection; an allergic reaction to local anesthetics, contrast, or steroids; dizziness; syncope; and hypertension can occur. A spinal cord injury is possible if the needle passes through a joint.

Intradiscal injection complications include pharynx or esophagus injury, discitis, hematoma, nerve root irritation, headache, pneumothorax (C7–T1 levels), vasovagal response (carotid body compression), and injectate allergic reaction [10].

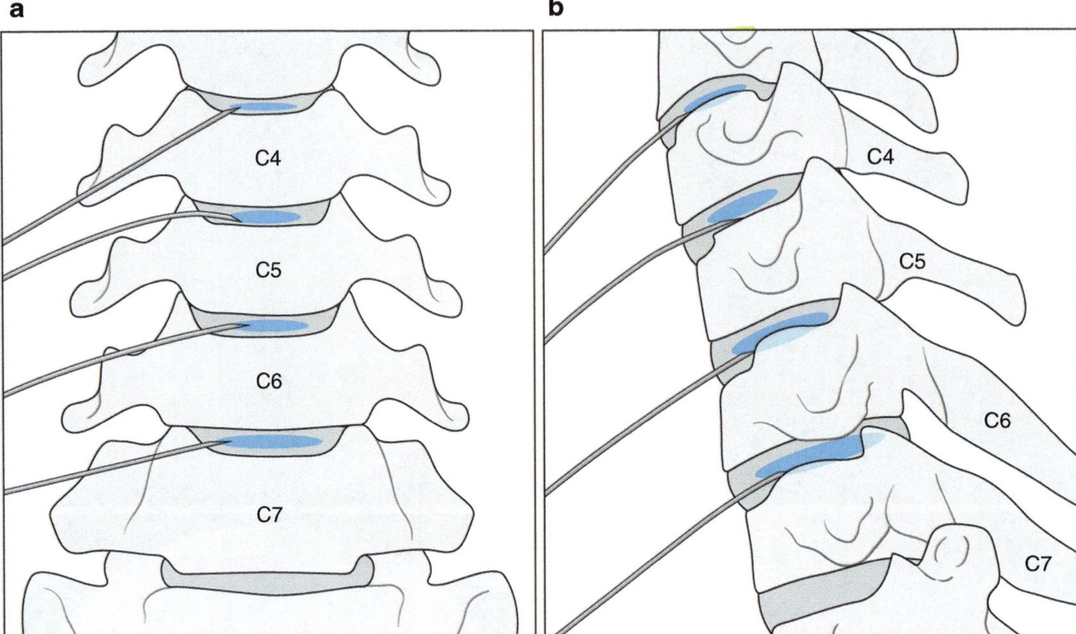

Fig. 5.6 Cervical intradiscal injection (*C4–C7*): anteroposterior (**a**) and lateral views (**b**) show the needle tips positioned in the centers of the intervertebral discs (Reproduced from Zaccagnino MP, Nedeljkovic SS. Lumbar, Thoracic, and Cervical Discography. Pain Medicine. 2017:249–256)

5.3 Thoracic Spine

5.3.1 Anatomical Considerations

The thoracic facet joints are nearly vertical and coronal in orientation and rotate towards the sagittal plane near the thoracolumbar junction. Each facet joint is angled between 65° and 75° from the transverse plane (Fig. 5.2) [8, 11].

Thoracic spine intradiscal procedures should be performed very carefully because the costovertebral junction nearly overlaps the pedicle in the sagittal plane, and the lung is nearby, lateral to the spine.

5.3.2 Techniques

5.3.2.1 Facet Injection [12]

1. The patient lies prone.
2. The C-arm is tilted caudally approximately 50° to 70°. The inferior articular process tip is targeted because the thoracic facet joints are not visible due to their steep angle (Fig. 5.7).
3. A 25-gauge, 3.5-inch spinal needle is inserted and advanced toward the target joint.
4. After the needle contacts the bone, it is withdrawn slightly, and its tip is inserted into the joint cavity.
5. After the needle is placed in the target joint, contrast is injected, and the needle tip position is confirmed by a circular contrast pattern on an arthrogram.
6. A mixture of local anesthetic and a steroid (approximately 1 mL) is carefully injected.

5.3.2.2 Intradiscal Injection [13]

1. The patient lies prone.
2. The C-arm is rotated ipsilaterally until the pedicle can be seen positioned over one-third of the vertebral body and a hyperlucent rectangle appears between the pedicle and the rib head (Fig. 5.8a).

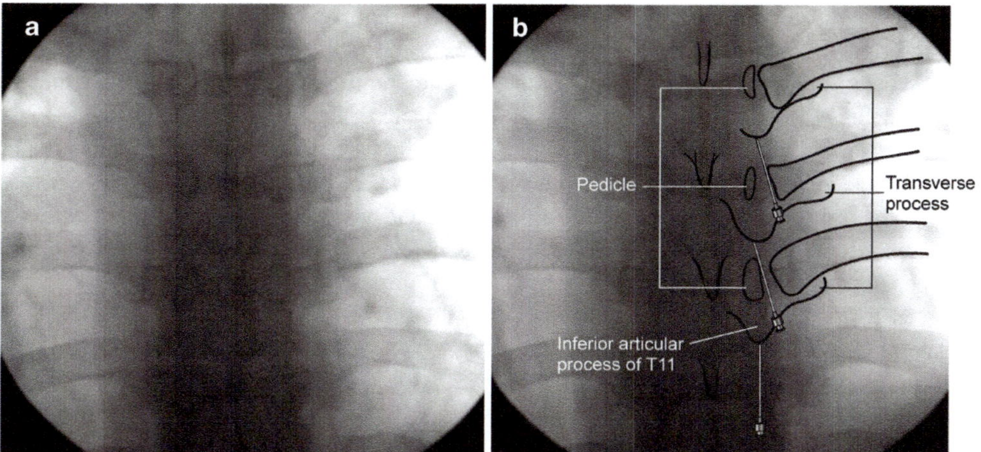

Fig. 5.7 Thoracic facet joint targeting: the facet joints are not visible due to their steep angle in the anteroposterior view (**a**). The needle is inserted into the inferior articular process (**b**) [12] (Reproduced from Rathmell JP. Atlas of image-guided intervention in regional anesthesia and pain medicine. 2nd ed. Philadelphia: Lippincott Williams & Wilkins, 2012. ISBN 978–1–60,831-704-2)

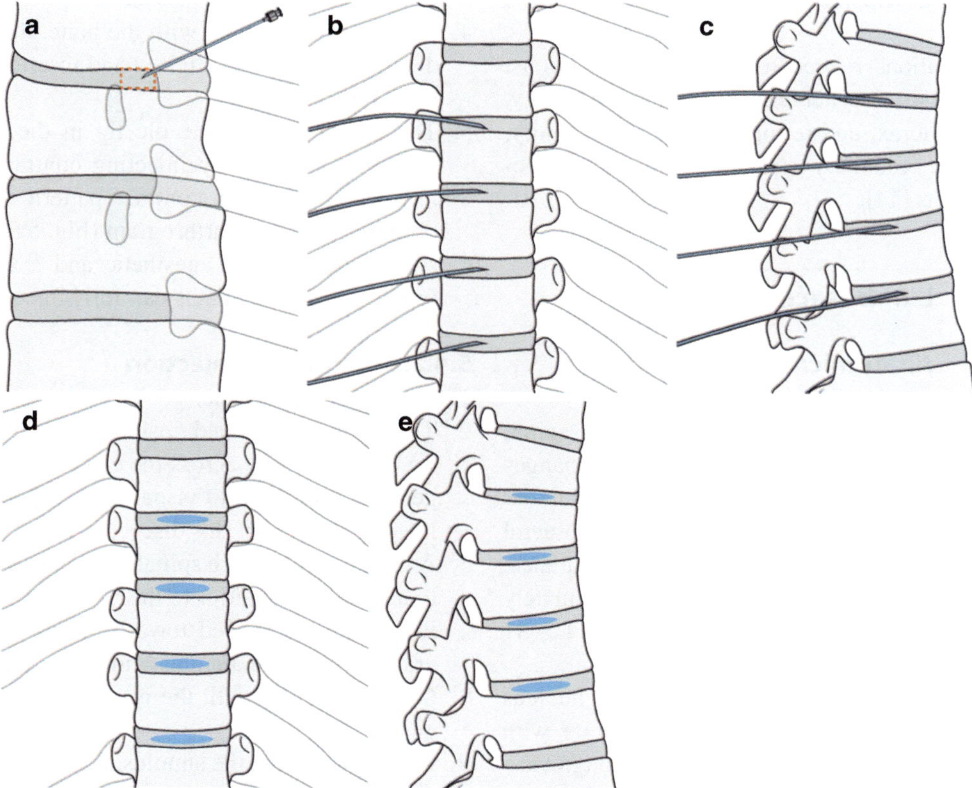

Fig. 5.8 Thoracic intradiscal injection: the spinal needle is inserted to lie over one-third of the vertebral body (**a**); anteroposterior (**b**) and lateral (**c**) views of the needle in the center of the intervertebral disc and anteroposterior (**d**) and lateral (**e**) views after intradiscal contrast injection [13] (Reproduced from Landers MH. Discography. In: Lennard TA, Walkowski S, Singla AK, Vivian DG, authors. Pain procedures in clinical practice. 3rd ed. Philadelphia: Elsevier Saunders; 2011. ISBN: 978–1–4160-3779-8)

3. A 25-gauge, 3.5-inch spinal needle is carefully inserted into the hyperlucent rectangle until it reaches the posterolateral aspect of the annulus in the AP and lateral C-arm views; the needle tip should be advanced between the borders of the lamina and the medial rib head to avoid the lung, which is just lateral to the rib head border (Fig. 5.8b, c).
4. After penetrating the annulus, the needle tip is advanced to the center of the IVD with AP and lateral C-arm guidance.
5. Contrast (approximately 0.5–1 mL) is injected, and a discogram is obtained to confirm the needle tip position (Fig. 5.8d, e).
6. A mixture of local anesthetic and a steroid or biologic agent (approximately 23 mL) is carefully injected.

5.3.3 Complications

Complications related to facet joint injections, including discitis, nerve root or spinal cord injury, pneumothorax, and retroperitoneal organ injury, can occur secondary to poor technique and injectate agents [14].

5.4 Lumbosacral Spine

5.4.1 Anatomical Considerations

The upper lumbar facet joints lie in the sagittal plane, and their orientation gradually changes from the coronal plane to oblique as the lumbar level increases. In the axial plane, the lumbosacral facet joints may have a flat or curved appearance. At the L2–L3 and L3–L4 levels, approximately 80% of the joints are curved, and at the L5–S1 level, 85% of the joints are flat [15, 16].

The IVDs are composed of the inner nucleus pulposus and outer AF. IVDs degenerate with age, and discogenic pain may occur through various pathophysiological mechanisms and usually occurs at lower lumbar levels. At the L5–S1 level, the spine is more tilted when compared to the other levels, and the IVD at this level is partly covered by the pelvis.

SI joints are paired c- or l-shaped joints. The ventral one-third of the joints making up each SI joint are true synovial joints, and the rest are intrinsic or extrinsic ligaments, such as the ventral, dorsal, and interosseous ligaments [17–19]. Because the lumbosacral plexus is near the superior and ventral part of each joint, referred pain can be produced in the proximal lower extremities.

5.4.2 Techniques

5.4.2.1 Facet Injection

1. The patient lies prone.
2. The C-arm is rotated ipsilaterally approximately 25° to 30°.
3. A 25-gauge, 3.5-inch spinal needle is advanced toward either the upper or lower end of the target joint (Fig. 5.9a).
4. After making contact with the bone, the needle tip is withdrawn slightly and inserted into the joint cavity.
5. The position of the needle tip in the target joint is confirmed by injecting contrast and identifying a linear contrast pattern in the oblique view on an arthrogram (Fig. 5.9).
6. A mixture of local anesthetic and a steroid (approximately 1 mL) is carefully injected.

5.4.2.2 Intradiscal Injection

1. The patient lies prone.
2. The C-arm is rotated ipsilaterally until the SAP is seen lying across the center of the target IVD and tilted to visualize the upper and lower endplates of this disc.
3. A 25-gauge, 3.5-inch spinal needle is inserted to a point just anterior to the SAP. The needle is carefully advanced toward the posterolateral aspect of the annulus with AP and lateral C-arm guidance until the needle contacts the annulus (Fig. 5.10a).
4. After penetrating the annulus, the needle tip is placed in the center of the IVD with AP and lateral C-arm guidance.
5. Contrast (approximately 1–2 mL) is injected, and a discogram is obtained to confirm the needle tip position (Fig. 5.10).

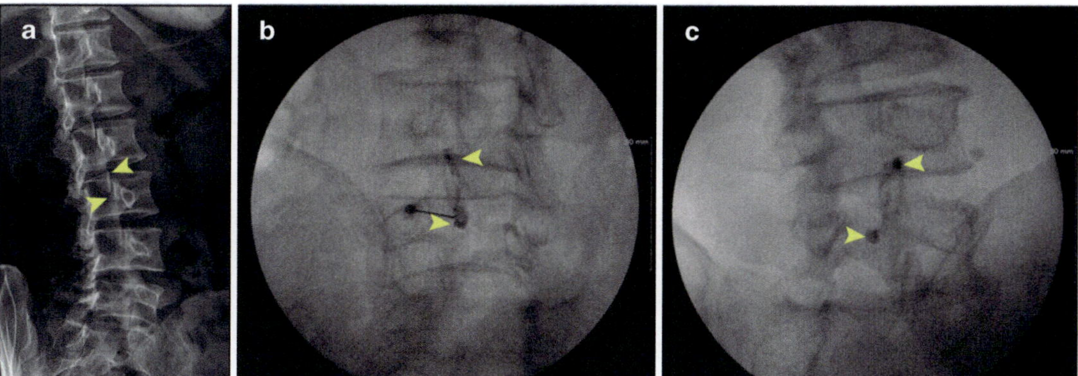

Fig. 5.9 Lumbar facet injection: the needle should be advanced toward the upper or lower end of the facet joint (L3–L4 shown here, *black arrows*) (**a**). An arthrogram shows an ipsilateral oblique view of the L4–L5 facet through the lower end of the joint (**b**). An arthrogram shows an ipsilateral oblique view of the L4–L5 facet through the upper end of the joint (**c**)

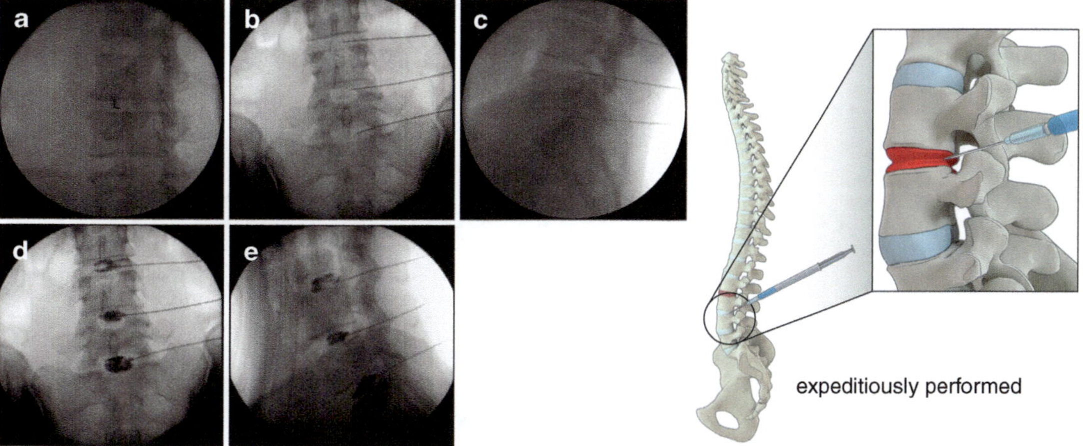

Fig. 5.10 Lumbosacral intervertebral discograms: a spinal needle is inserted into a point just anterior to the SAP until it contacts the annulus (**a**); the needle tip is seen at the center of the intervertebral disc in the anteroposterior (**b**) and lateral (**c**) views, and the discograms show the anteroposterior (**d**) and lateral views (**e**) of levels L3–L4, L4–L5, and L5–S1

6. A mixture of local anesthetic and a steroid or regenerative agent (approximately 2–3 mL) is carefully injected.

5.4.2.3 Sacroiliac Joint Injection: Upper One-Third Approach

1. The patient lies prone.
2. The C-arm is rotated contralaterally about 25° to 40°.
3. The wedge shape between the medial border of the ilium and the lateral border of the sacral ala is identified.
4. A 25-gauge, 3.5-inch spinal needle is inserted into the wedge shape.
5. After the needle contacts the bone, the C-arm is rotated to the AP view.
6. The needle is then advanced laterally and inferiorly into the SI joint.
7. When the needle is in the target joint, contrast is injected, and the needle tip position is confirmed by arthrograms showing a linear contrast pattern in AP and contralateral views and a c-shape contrast pattern in the ipsilateral view (Fig. 5.11).

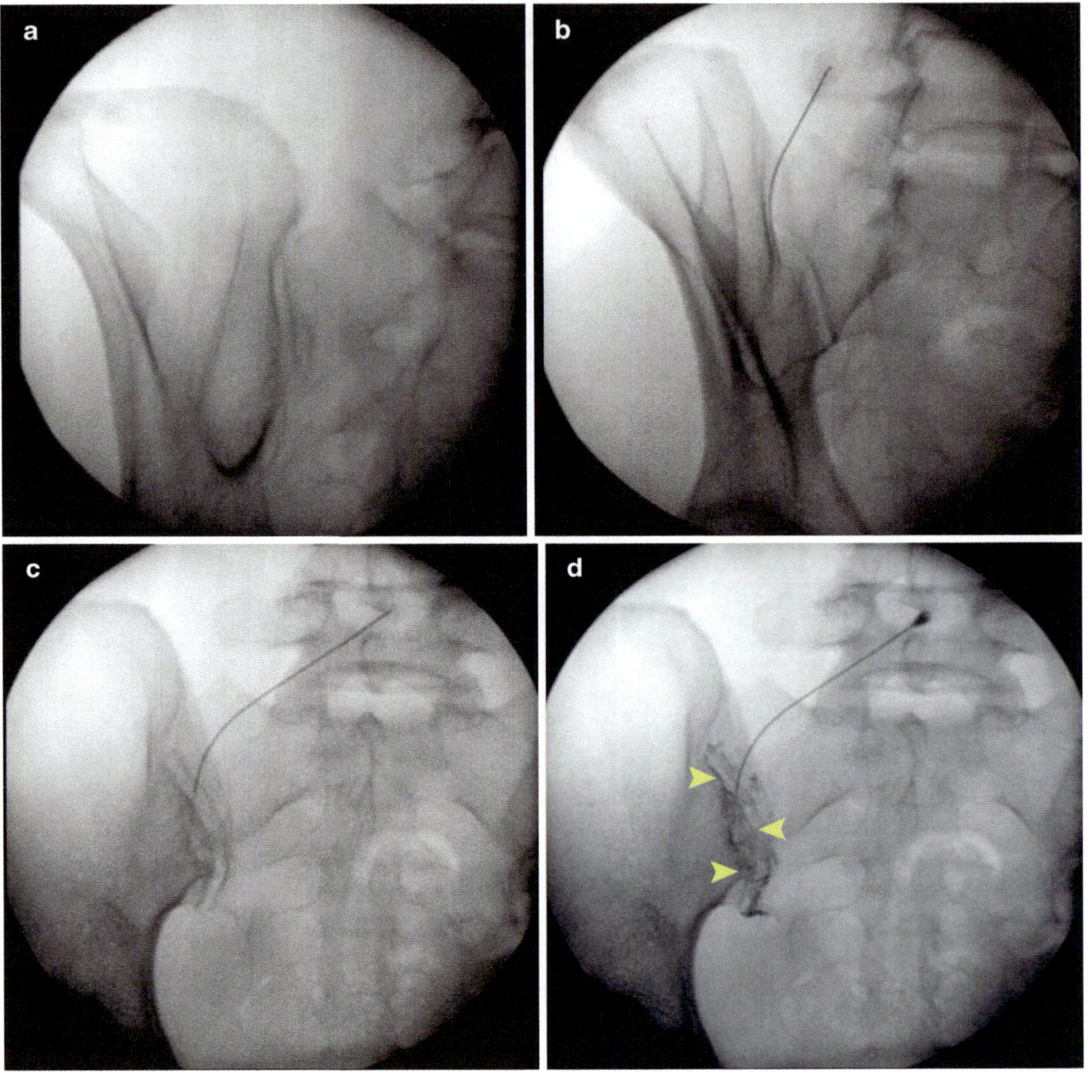

Fig. 5.11 Sacroiliac joint injection using the upper one-third approach: the wedge-shaped space between the medial border of the ilium and the lateral border of the sacral ala (**a**); the needle passes through the wedge-shaped space to the sacroiliac joint space (**b**); needle tip placement in the joint space in the anteroposterior view (**c**); and an arthrogram in the anteroposterior view (**d**)

8. A mixture of local anesthetic and a steroid (approximately 2 mL) is injected carefully.
9. Before an interosseous ligament injection, the needle is withdrawn cranially, contrast is injected, and the needle tip position is confirmed by an arthrogram showing a cloud-like pattern; the injectate described above (2 mL) is then carefully injected.

5.4.2.4 Sacroiliac Joint Injection: Lower One-Third Approach

1. The patient lies prone.
2. The C-arm is rotated contralaterally about 5°, and the area where the anterior and posterior joints overlap at the lower end of the SI joint is identified.

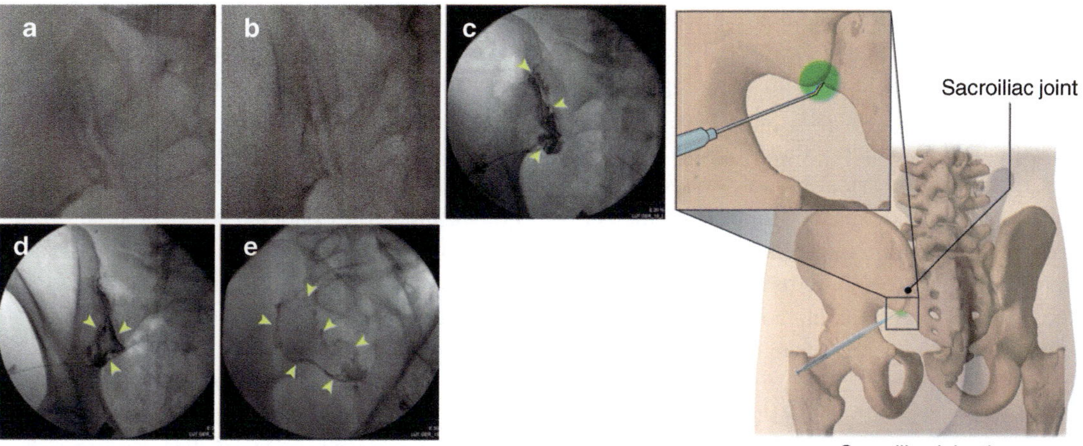

Fig. 5.12 Sacroiliac joint injection using the lower one-third approach: the anteroposterior view shows the separately positioned posterior (medial) and anterior (lateral) joints (**a**); the contralateral rotation view at 5° shows the two joints overlapping (**b**); an arthrogram shows a linear contrast pattern in anteroposterior (**c**) and contralateral (**d**) views and a c-shape in the ipsilateral view (**e**)

3. A 25-gauge, 3.5-inch spinal needle is inserted and advanced to the target.
4. After the needle contacts the bone, it is withdrawn slightly and inserted into the joint cavity.
5. When the needle is in the target joint, contrast is injected, and the needle tip position is confirmed by arthrograms showing a linear contrast pattern in AP and contralateral views and a c-shaped pattern in the ipsilateral view (Fig. 5.12).
6. A mixture of local anesthetic and a steroid (approximately 2 mL) is carefully injected.

5.4.3 Complications

Intra-articular facet and SI joint injection-associated complications are uncommon. Bleeding, infection, and an allergic reaction to the injectate can occur. After interosseous ligament injection, transient proximal leg weakness due to extravasation of the local anesthetic to the lumbosacral plexus can also occur.

Intradiscal injection-related complications are also uncommon and include discitis, disc penetration, needle misplacement, nausea, headache, and an allergic reaction to the injectate.

5.5 Discussion

5.5.1 Cervical Spine

Steroids and local anesthetics have anti-inflammatory effects and cause pain relief by stabilizing neural membranes. Both also have an anesthetic effect on small non-myelinated nociceptive C-fibers and inhibit leukocyte activity [20–23]. These agents are used to treat pain secondary to inflammation, such as the pain of osteoarthritis.

Cervical facet joint steroid injections have been used to treat cervical facet joint-related pain. In Roy et al.'s study of 39 cases of fluoroscopy-guided cervical facet joint infiltration, 91% of the patients experienced symptom relief [24]. However, in a more recent study, level IV evidence demonstrated the effectiveness of cervical facet intra-articular injection for long-term improvement in patients with chronic cervical facet joint pain [25]. This result indicates that inflammation is not a major cause of chronic facet joint pain.

Upper cervical facet joint pathology induces headaches as well as neck pain. This effect may be explained by a theory that suggests headaches can result from cervical pathology secondary to the convergence of sensory input from the cervical structures within the spinal nucleus of the trigeminal nerve [26]. Dreyfuss et al. reported that the lateral atlanto-axial and atlanto-occipital joints are pain generators capable of causing neck pain and headaches [27].

Glémarec J et al. studied the effect of lateral atlanto-axial joint glucocorticoid injection and found that patients experienced a mean pain scale score decrease of approximately 52.3%, and this pain relief lasted about 8.1 months [28]. Lee et al. investigated the effect of atlanto-occipital joint injection in patients with chronic refractory neck pain or headaches. The patients had a limited range of lateral bending with rotation at the atlanto-occipital joint and pain relief of at least 50% after diagnostic injections. Two months after therapeutic injections, the pain scores of headache and neck pain decreased from 5.64 and 5.70 to 0.64 and 2.30, respectively [29]. Intradiscal injections are typically employed for diagnostic purposes but are occasionally used for treatment.

In Wilkinson et al.'s study of 21 injections performed in 14 patients with cervical disc disease and discogenic neck or arm pain, 65% of patients experienced pain relief that lasted 1 month. However, this effect persisted in only 15% after 3 months [30].

5.5.2 Thoracic Spine

The causes of thoracic spine pain have no specific radiologic or physical examination characteristics or other diagnostic features. Therefore, patients with thoracic spine pain require a diagnostic thoracic facet or medial branch block to identify thoracic facet joint pain and rule out discogenic pain. Although there is no evidence available indicating the long-term effectiveness of thoracic intra-articular facet joint injections [31], thoracic facet joint intra-articular steroid injection is sometimes used for middle-back pain.

In a recent study, Manchikanti et al. investigated the effects of thoracic facet and medial branch blocks. In patients whose source of pain was confirmed using medial branch blocks or intra-articular facet injections, approximately 70% had pain relief greater than 50% for 2 years following a therapeutic procedure [32].

The prevalence of discogenic thoracic pain is unknown. Further, the evidence supporting the use of thoracic provocation discography is limited because of the test's potential for false-positive responses and the inability to rule out other sources of pain [33].

5.5.3 Lumbosacral Spine

Carette et al. reported the effectiveness of lumbosacral intra-articular steroid injections for the treatment of lumbosacral facet joint pain that was previously confirmed by diagnostic injections [34]. Since then, this procedure has been widely used. There is level III evidence of long-term improvement after lumbosacral intra-articular injection [25], and the procedure may be more useful in circumstances where short-term relief is needed or adjuvant therapy (e.g., physiotherapy) is provided [35].

The results of intradiscal steroid injections are variable [36–39]. The rationale for steroid use is that steroids function as phospholipase A2 inhibitors in the inflammatory pathway [38, 39]. Further, patients with discogenic pain have higher levels of proinflammatory mediators in their disc tissue than patients with sciatica. Similarly, patients with Modic type I endplate changes have higher levels of proinflammatory mediators than do patients with Modic type II or III changes [40, 41].

Buttermann reported that intradiscal steroid injections effectively reduce pain in patients with inflammatory endplate changes on magnetic resonance imaging (MRI), and Fayad et al. also reported successful pain management 1 month after intradiscal steroid injection in patients with Modic type I or II endplate abnormalities with predominantly edematous changes [42, 43].

Platelet-rich plasma (PRP) is used as a biologic agent for the treatment of discogenic pain. Tuakli-Wosornu et al. performed a prospective, double-blind RCT of PRP for the treatment of pain related to degenerative disc disease. A total of 47 participants were analyzed, and statistically significant improvements in pain, function, and patient satisfaction were seen in participants who received intradiscal PRP compared with controls [44]. After PRP administration, endothelial growth factor, platelet-derived growth factor, vascular endothelial growth factor, and basic fibroblast growth factor stimulate the production of collagen types I and III, angiogenesis, cell proliferation, cytoprotection, and stem cell proliferation and differentiation and influence the production of collagen, a proteoglycan [45].

The evidence supporting the use of intra-articular and peri-articular injections for SI joint treatment is limited [14]. The therapeutic effects of the various injection methods (e.g., upper and lower one-third approaches [46] and C-arm- or ultrasonography-guided) are nearly the same [47].

References

1. Boswell MV, Colson JD, Sehgal N, Dunbar EE, Epter R. A systematic review of therapeutic facet joint interventions in chronic spinal pain. Pain Physician. 2007;10:229–53.
2. Yin W, Bogduk N. The nature of neck pain in a private pain clinic in the United States. Pain Med. 2008;9:196–203.
3. Thawrani DP, Agabegi SS, Asghar F. Diagnosing sacroiliac joint pain. J Am Acad Orthop Surg. 2019;27:85–93.
4. Ohtori S, Inoue G, Miyagi M, Takahashi K. Pathomechanisms of discogenic low back pain in humans and animal models. Spine J. 2015;15:1347–55.
5. Standing S, Borely NR, Collins P, Crossman AR, Gatzoulis MA, Healy GC, et al. Gray's anatomy: the anatomical basis of clinical practice. 40th ed. London: Churchill Livingstone; 2008. ISBN: 978-0-8089-2371-8.
6. Lu J, Ebraheim NA. Anatomic considerations of C2 nerve root ganglion. Spine (Phila Pa 1976). 1998;15:649–52.
7. Mercer S, Bogduk N. The ligaments and annulus fibrosis of human adult cervical intervertebral discs. Spine (Phila Pa 1976). 1999;24:619–28.
8. Beyaz SG, Sayhan H. Six-month results of cervical intradiscal oxygen-ozone mixture therapy on patients with neck pain: preliminary findings. Pain Physician. 2018;21:E449–56.
9. Panjabi MM, Oxland T, Takata K, Goel V, Duranceau J, Krag M. Articular facets of the human spine. Quantitative three-dimensional anatomy. Spine (Phila Pa 1976). 1993;18:1298–310.
10. Moringlane JR, Koch R, Schäfer H, Ostertag CB. Experimental radiofrequency (RF) coagulation with computer-based on line monitoring of temperature and power. Acta Neurochir. 1989;96:126–31.
11. Ebraheim NA, Xu R, Ahmad M, Yeasting RA. The quantitative anatomy of the thoracic facet and the posterior projection of its inferior facet. Spine (Phila Pa 1976). 1997;22:1811–7.
12. Rathmell JP. Atlas of image-guided intervention in regional anesthesia and pain medicine. 2nd ed. Philadelphia: Lippincott Williams & Wilkins; 2012. ISBN: 978-1-60831-704-2.
13. Landers MH. Discography. In: Lennard TA, Walkowski S, Singla AK, Vivian DG, editors. Pain procedures in clinical practice. 3rd ed. Philadelphia: Elsevier Saunders; 2011. ISBN: 978-1-4160-3779-8.
14. Manchikanti L, Abdi S, Atluri S, Benyamin RM, Boswell MV, Buenaventura RM, et al. An update of comprehensive evidence-based guidelines for interventional techniques in chronic spinal pain. Part II: guidance and recommendations. Pain Physician. 2013;16(2 Suppl):S49–283.
15. Bogduk N. Clinical anatomy of the lumbar spine and sacrum. 3rd ed. New York: Churchill Livingstone; 1997.
16. Raj PP, Lou L, Erdine S, Peter S, Stoats PS, Steven D, et al. International pain management: image-guided procedures. 2nd ed. Philadelphia: Saunders; 2008. ISBN: 978-1-4160-3844-3.
17. Puhakka KB, Melsen F, Jurik AG, Boel LW, Vesterby A, Egund N. MR imaging of the normal sacroiliac joint with correlation to histology. Skelet Radiol. 2004;33:15–28.
18. Cohen SP. Sacroiliac joint pain: a comprehensive review of anatomy, diagnosis, and treatment. Anesth Analg. 2005;101:1440–53.
19. Steinke H, Hammer N, Slowik V, Stadler J, Josten C, Böhme J, et al. Novel insights into the sacroiliac joint ligaments. Spine (Phila Pa 1976). 2010;35:257–63.
20. Pobiel RS, Schellhas KP, Eklund JA, Golden MJ, Johnson BA, Chopra S, et al. Selective cervical nerve root blockade: prospective study of immediate and longer term complications. AJNR Am J Neuroradiol. 2009;30:507–11.

21. Slipman CW, Lipetz JS, Jackson HB, Rogers DP, Vresilovic EJ. Therapeutic selective nerve root block in the nonsurgical treatment of atraumatic cervical spondylotic radicular pain: a retrospective analysis with independent clinical review. Arch Phys Med Rehabil. 2000;81:741–6.
22. Anderberg L, Annertz M, Persson L, Brandt L, Säveland H. Transforaminal steroid injections for the treatment of cervical radiculopathy: a prospective and randomised study. Eur Spine J. 2007;16:321–8.
23. Yabuki S, Kawaguchi Y, Nordborg C, Kikuchi S, Rydevik B, Olmarker K. Effects of lidocaine on nucleus pulposus-induced nerve root injury. A neurophysiologic and histologic study of the pig cauda equina. Spine (Phila Pa 1976). 1998;23:2383–9.
24. Roy DF, Fleury J, Fontaine SB, Dussault RG. Clinical evaluation of cervical facet joint infiltration. Can Assoc Radiol J. 1988;39:118–20.
25. Manchikanti L, Kaye AD, Boswell MV, Bakshi S, Gharibo CG, Grami V, et al. A systematic review and best evidence synthesis of the effectiveness of therapeutic facet joint interventions in managing chronic spinal pain. Pain Physician. 2015;18:E535–82.
26. Haldeman S, Dagenais S. Cervicogenic headaches: a critical review. Spine J. 2001;1:31–46.
27. Dreyfuss P, Michaelsen M, Fletcher D. Atlanto-occipital and lateral atlanto-axial joint pain patterns. Spine (Phila Pa 1976). 1994;19:1125–31.
28. Glémarec J, Guillot P, Laborie Y, Berthelot JM, Prost A, Maugars Y. Intraarticular glucocorticosteroid injection into the lateral atlantoaxial joint under fluoroscopic control. A retrospective comparative study in patients with mechanical and inflammatory disorders. Joint Bone Spine. 2000;67:54–61.
29. Lee DG, Cho YW, Jang SH, Son SM, Kim GJ, Ahn SH. Effectiveness of intra-articular steroid injection for atlanto-occipital joint pain. Pain Med. 2015;16:1077–82.
30. Wilkinson HA, Schuman N. Intradiscal corticosteroids in the treatment of lumbar and cervical disc problems. Spine (Phila Pa 1976). 1980;5:385–9.
31. Manchikanti L, Boswell MV, Datta S, Fellows B, Abdi S, Singh V, et al. Comprehensive review of therapeutic interventions in managing chronic spinal pain. Pain Physician. 2009;12:E123–98.
32. Manchikanti L, Boswell MV, Singh V, Pampati V, Damron KS, Beyer CD. Prevalence of facet joint pain in chronic spinal pain of cervical, thoracic, and lumbar regions. BMC Musculoskelet Disord. 2004;5:15.
33. Merskey H, Bogduk N. Thoracic discogenic pain. In: International Association for the Study of Pain. Classification of chronic pain. Descriptions of chronic pain syndromes and definition of pain terms. 2nd ed. Seattle: IASP Press; 1994, p. 116.
34. Carette S, Marcoux S, Truchon R, Grondin C, Gagnon J, Allard Y, et al. A controlled trial of corticosteroid injections into facet joints for chronic low back pain. New Engl J Med. 1991;325:1002–7.
35. Chambers H. Physiotherapy and lumbar facet joint injections as a combination treatment for chronic low back pain. A narrative review of lumbar facet joint injections, lumbar spinal mobilizations, soft tissue massage and lower back mobility exercises. Musculoskeletal Care. 2013;11:106–20.
36. Feffer HL. Therapeutic intradiscal hydrocortisone. A long-term study. Clin Orthop Relat Res. 1969;67:100–4.
37. Graham CE. Chemonucleolysis. A preliminary report on a double blind study comparing chemonucleolysis and intradiscal administration of hydrocortisone in the treatment of backache and sciatica. Orthop Clin North Am. 1975;6:259–63.
38. Khot A, Bowditch M, Powell J, Sharp D. The use of intradiscal steroid therapy for lumbar spinal discogenic pain: a randomized controlled trial. Spine (Phila Pa 1976). 2004;29:833–6.
39. Simmons JW, McMillin JN, Emery SF, Kimmich SJ. Intradiscal steroids. A prospective double-blind clinical trial Spine (Phila Pa 1976). 1992;17(6 Suppl):S172–5.
40. Burke JG, Watson RW, McCormack D, Dowling FE, Walsh MG, Fitzpatrick JM. Intervertebral discs which cause low back pain secrete high levels of proinflammatory mediators. Bone Joint Surg Br. 2002;84:196–201.
41. Ohtori S, Inoue G, Ito T, Koshi T, Ozawa T, Doya H, et al. Tumor necrosis factor-immunoreactive cells and PGP 9.5-immunoreactive nerve fibers in vertebral endplates of patients with discogenic low back pain and Modic type 1 or type 2 changes on MRI. Spine (Phila Pa 1976). 2006;31:1026–31.
42. Fayad F, Lefevre-Colau MM, Rannou F, Quintero N, Nys A, Macé Y, et al. Relation of inflammatory modic changes to intradiscal steroid injection outcome in chronic low back pain. Eur Spine J. 2007;16:925–31.
43. Buttermann GR. The effect of spinal steroid injections for degenerative disc disease. Spine J. 2004;4:495–505.
44. Tuakli-Wosornu YA, Terry A, Boachie-Adjei K, Harrison JR, Gribbin CK, LaSalle EE, et al. Lumbar intradiskal platelet-rich plasma (PRP) injections: a prospective, double-blind, randomized controlled study. PM R. 2016;8:1–10.
45. Navani A, Manchikanti L, Albers SL, Latchaw RE, Sanapati J, Kaye AD, et al. Responsible, safe, and effective use of biologics in the management of low back pain: American Society of Interventional Pain Physicians (ASIPP) guidelines. Pain Physician. 2019;22(1S):S1–74.
46. Hong SH, Chung H, Lee CH, Kim YH. A prospective randomized noninferiority trial comparing upper and lower one-third joint approaches for sacroiliac joint injections. Pain Physician. 2018;21:251–8.
47. Soneji N, Bhatia A, Seib R, Tumber P, Dissanayake M, Peng PW. Comparison of fluoroscopy and ultrasound guidance for sacroiliac joint injection in patients with chronic low back pain. Pain Pract. 2016;16:537–44.

Part II

Particulars

6 Percutaneous Epidural Neuroplasty

Pyung Goo Cho, Gyu Yeul Ji, and Dong Ah Shin

6.1 Introduction

Percutaneous epidural neuroplasty (PEN) is a minimally invasive spine management technique. It is referred to as percutaneous epidural neurolysis, Racz procedure, or the percutaneous epidural adhesiolysis. PEN plays a role in epidural scar dissolution, target drug delivery, ventral space drug injection, and the nerve decompression [1, 2]. After inserting a catheter into the target area where adhesions are visible on epidural examination, adhesiolysis is performed. A soft or navigable catheter system can be used to successfully advance the catheter to the target site in the epidural space. The adhesiolysis technique consists of mechanical dissolution using a catheter, chemical dissolution using hyaluronidase, and hydrostatic pressure dissolution using physiological saline and a contrast medium. The navigable catheter is more useful for mechanical lysis because the catheter tip can be moved from side to side.

PEN is a proven treatment for chronic pain in patients with post spinal surgery syndrome [3–7]. It has also been proven effective in cases of herniated lumbar disc with radiating pain and spinal stenosis [2, 4, 8, 9].

P. G. Cho
Department of Neurosurgery, Ajou University Medical Center, Suwon-si, Republic of Korea

G. Y. Ji (✉)
Department of Neurosurgery, Yonsei Hana Hospital, Gimpo-si, Republic of Korea

D. A. Shin
Department of Neurosurgery, Yonsei University Severance Hospital, Seoul, Republic of Korea

6.2 History of Percutaneous Epidural Neuroplasty

In 1989, Gabor Racz named as percutaneous epidural adhesiolysis and developed and advanced it. Racz suggested that 60% of symptomatic recurrences after spinal surgery are caused by epidural adhesions. The purpose of this treatment was to remove fibrous epidural adhesions in patients with failed back spine surgery (FBSS) syndrome [10–12]. Postoperative adhesions are tenacious, and microscopic adhesions are also found in patients with an intervertebral hernia or chronic back pain [13, 14]. In 1999, Racz renamed the procedure PEN and extended its indications to patients with post-spinal surgery syndrome as well as patients with herniated lumbar disc (HLD), spinal stenosis and chronic low back pain syndrome [11].

6.3 Indications

PEN has been proposed as an effective method for patients with FBSS syndrome, HLD, or chronic back pain who do not respond to conventional conservative treatment [3–7, 9]. After

S.-H. Lee (ed.), *Minimally Invasive Spine Interventions*,
https://doi.org/10.1007/978-981-16-9547-6_6

applying the rigorous evaluation criteria of the United States Preventative Services Task Force, there is good evidence to indicate that PEN is effective treatment method in patients with FBSS syndrome or spinal stenosis [15]. However, evidence indicating that adhesiolysis is effective for HLD or chronic spinal pain diagnosed using the same criteria is still limited [15]. Contraindications to PEN include local or systemic infection, coagulopathy, patient refusal, syrinx formation, and arachnoiditis.

6.4 Surgical Technique

Step 1 Preoperative Preparation

Informed consent should be obtained before conducting PEN. The PEN procedure should be performed in an operating room that maintains aseptic conditions and should be performed by a medical professional with specialized knowledge. It is recommended to inject prophylactic antibiotics before the procedure.

Step 2 Sacral Hiatus Puncture

The patient is placed in the prone position with a pillow under the abdomen to minimize lumbar lordosis. First, make the sterile preparation and draping, and then the sacral hiatus is identified by palpation. This step can be made easier by fluoroscopy guidance. After injecting local anesthetic (1% or 2% lidocaine) into the skin of this area, wait for about 5 min until anesthesia is achieved. The skin is incision with an 15-blade, and a 15-gauge Tuohy needle is inserted at a 45° angle into the sacral foramen and fluoroscopically introduced into the spinal canal (Fig. 6.1). Tuohy needles come in a variety of shapes and sizes.

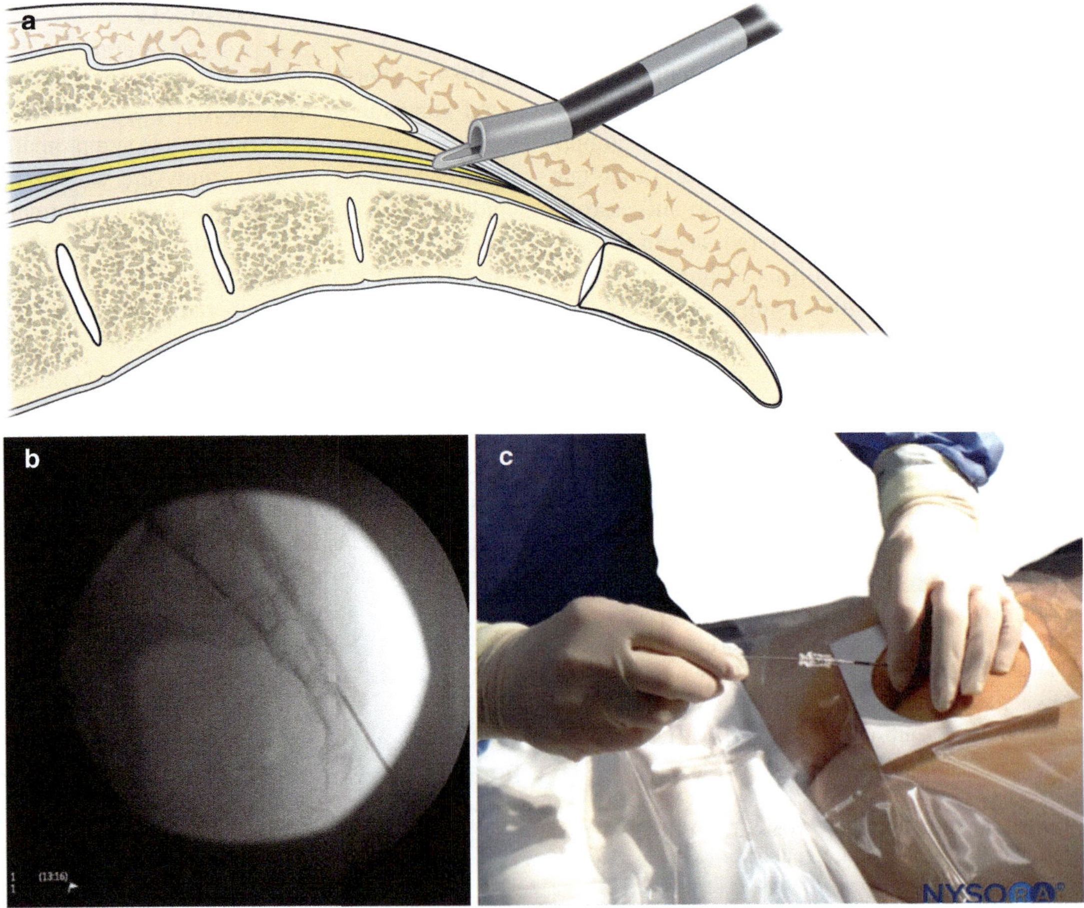

Fig. 6.1 (**a**) 15-gauge Tuohy needle is inserted through the sacral hiatus. (**b**) Fluoroscopic image of Tuohy needle into the sacral hiatus. (**c**) Insertion a soft catheter into this Tuohy needle

When the needle is through the hiatus, the angle of the needle is dropped to approximately 30°, and the needle is advanced. Depending on the shape of the sacrum, the operator may need to lay the needle down. The posterior edge of the distal opening of most Tuohy needles has a non-cutting surface. However, some needles have a cutting surface, which could easily shear the catheter. A properly placed needle will be inside the caudal canal below the level of the S3 foramen on AP and lateral fluoroscopic images because the sacral dura sac is typically located above the S3 vertebral body. If the needle is raised to the S3 level or higher, dura may be punctured, so be careful.

Step 3 Epidurogram

After placing the needle, the operator must check whether negative pressure is maintained through aspiration. This is because, if a contrast agent or drug is incorrectly injected into the subarachnoid space, the patient may have adverse events such as seizures or death. After the needle is placed in epidural space, an epidurogram is performed using a non-ionic, water-soluble contrast agent (iohexol). The contrast agent is slowly injected, and the epidurogram is evaluated for filling defects. A normal epidurogram will have a "Christmas tree" pattern with the central canal being the trunk and the outline of the nerve roots making up the branches (Fig. 6.2). If vascular uptake is observed, the needle needs to be repositioned. After passing the S3 level, the needle tip should cross the midline of the sacrum toward the side of the radiculopathy.

Step 4 Soft Catheter Advancement

After turning the bevel of the guide needle toward the ventral, insert a soft catheter into this guide needle (Fig. 6.1c). Considering the angle of the sacrum, to enter the ventral of the dura, a 2.5 cm part of the catheter string must be bent by 30° (Fig. 6.3a). Under AP fluoroscopy guidance, advance the tip of the catheter along the ventral aspect of the dura to reach the lesion. It is easier to reach the lesion by advancing with gentle rotation (Fig. 6.4). It is difficult for the catheter to advance from the ventral of the dura of the sacrum to the midline. Ideally, the catheter tip

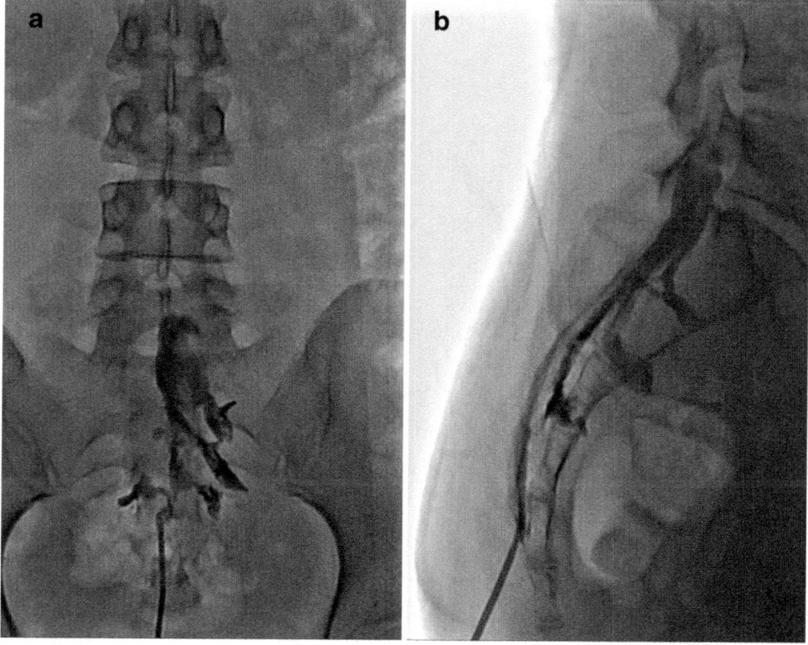

Fig. 6.2 An epidurogram shows an abnormal, asymmetric "tree" pattern after injection of iohexol (3 mL), possibly secondary to microscopic adhesions. (**a**) anteroposterior image in X-ray. (**b**) lateral image in X-ray

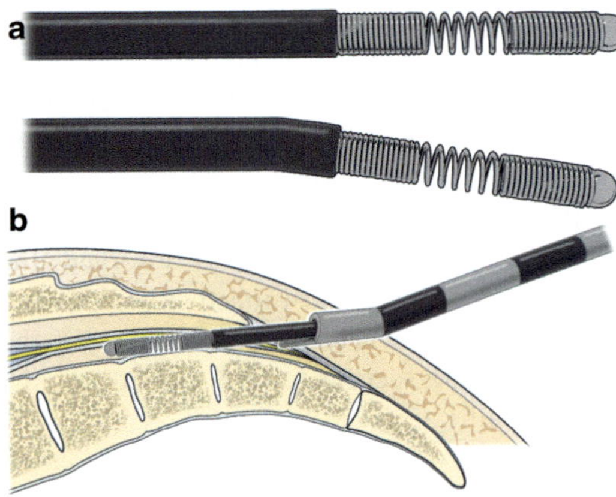

Fig. 6.3 A soft catheter (Tun-L-XL, Epimed, Dallas, TX, USA) with a bent distal tip: (**a**) the angle is typically 30° and 2.5 cm from the catheter tip. (**b**) the catheter is navigated through the needle and advanced to the target level

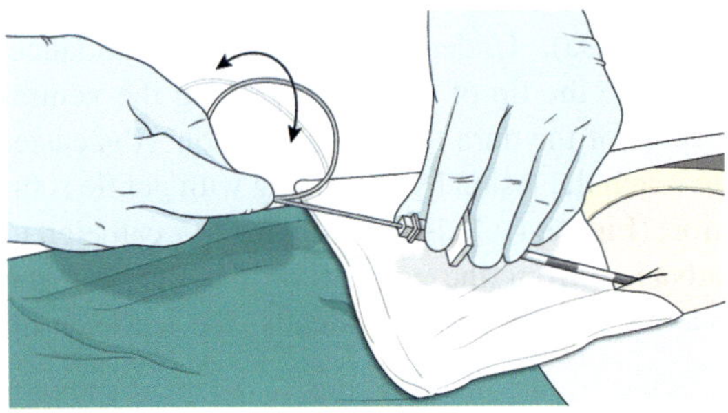

Fig. 6.4 A notch facilitates catheter steering

should be positioned to the midportion of the pedicle shadow in the AP projection, and the catheter tip in the lateral projection should be in the ventral epidural space (Fig. 6.5).

Step 5 Navigable Catheter Advancement

Navigable catheters have two major advantages over soft catheters. First, it is possible to change the navigable catheter's direction without bending the tip preoperatively. Second, navigable catheters are typically thicker and harder and can be used to lyse adhesions more forcefully (Fig. 6.6). An epidurogram is performed before the catheter is introduced, and it can be used to direct further catheter advancement. This process is identical to that used when working with a soft catheter system (Fig. 6.2). If the target is the DRG or neural foramen, the catheter tip should be directed toward the level below the target level. For example, to reach the L4–L5 neural foramen, the catheter must be directed toward the L5–S1 level. There are two ways to reach the ventral epidural space. The first is to enter the ventral epidural space at the S2–S3 level. This method requires passing instruments through the ventral epidural space throughout the procedure; therefore, the patient may experience significant pain. The second method is to approach the dor-

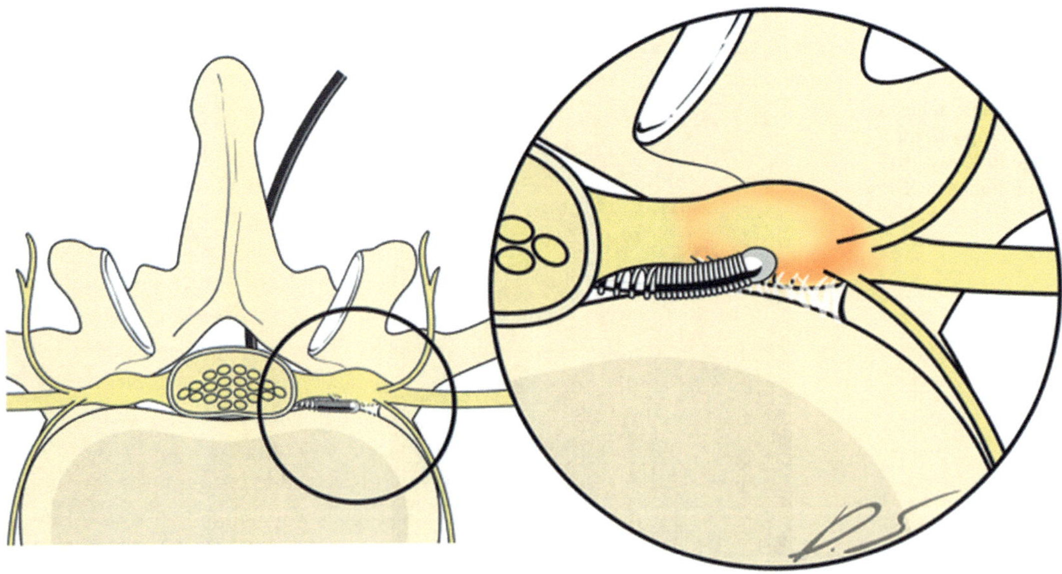

Fig. 6.5 The final catheter tip position in the case of foraminal stenosis; the target lesion is usually located in the ventral epidural space

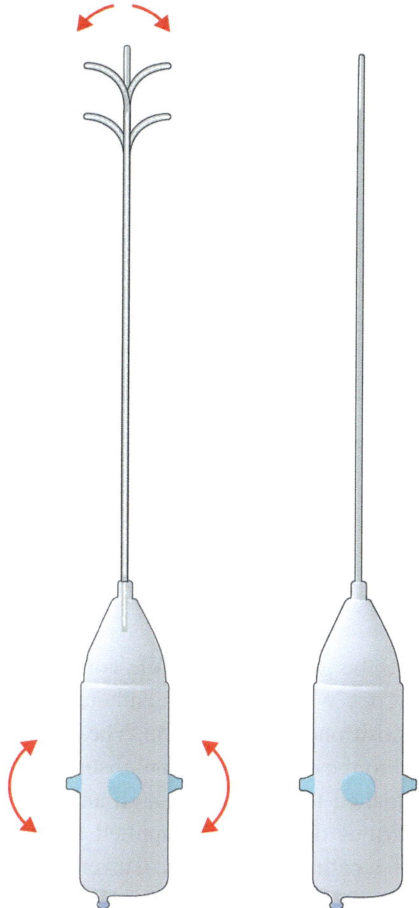

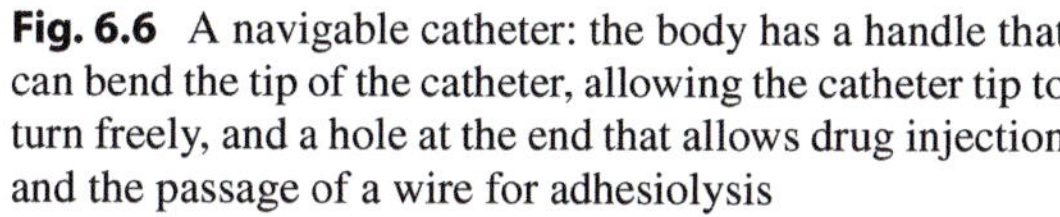

Fig. 6.6 A navigable catheter: the body has a handle that can bend the tip of the catheter, allowing the catheter tip to turn freely, and a hole at the end that allows drug injection and the passage of a wire for adhesiolysis

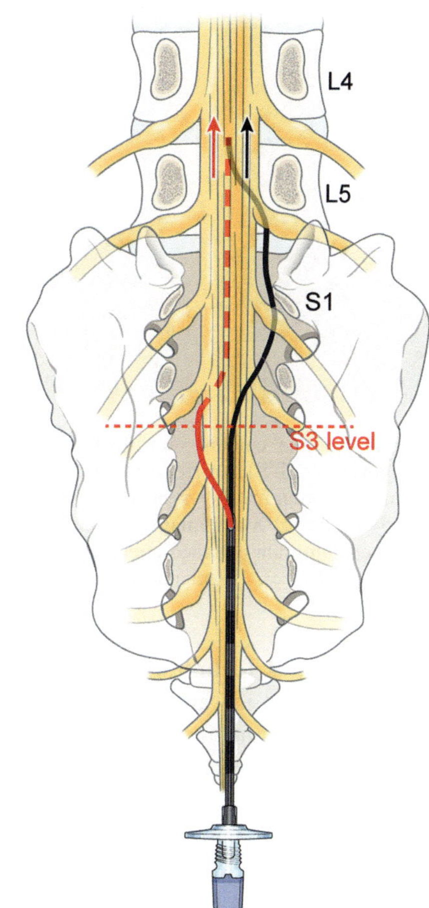

Fig. 6.7 Two approaches to catheter placement within the ventral epidural space: approach from the S2–S3 level (this method irritates the sinuvertebral nerve, resulting in significant pain) [1]; approach from the dorsal epidural space one level below the target level; here, the ventral epidural space is entered from the neural foramen to access the midline ventral space [2]

sal epidural space at the level below the target level and then enter the ventral epidural space from the neural foramen to access the midline ventral space (Fig. 6.7). The technique causes minimal pain, but learning how to successfully guide the catheter into the ventral space at the neural foramen takes time.

Because navigable catheters are typically thicker and harder than soft catheters, the procedures in which they are used can be more painful than the soft catheter procedures. There are ways to reduce procedure-related pain, including gentle catheter manipulation, a contrast-lidocaine mix (3:2), and the dorsal approach to the destination. Navigable catheters have other disadvantages; they cannot be changed to continuous injection after adhesiolysis or neuroplasty, and because they are hard, they can easily cause a dura laceration. The features of an effective catheter are as follows:

1. The catheter's distal end is bent, and the remaining part is straight.
2. The angle at the distal end should be over 180°.
3. The surface of the catheter is smooth and glides over the tissue.
4. The catheter handle is ergonomic.
5. The length of the catheter is long enough to reach the L2–L3 level.

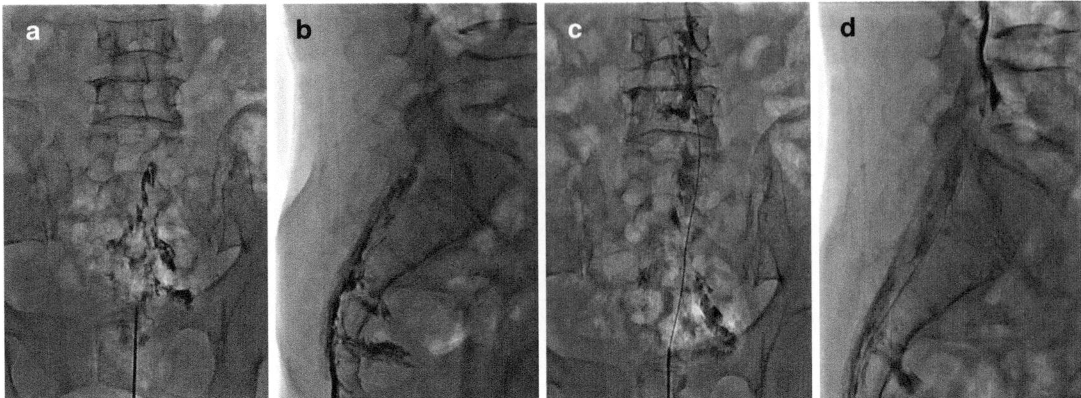

Fig. 6.8 (**a**) Routine epidurogram shows no contrast above the level of L5–S1, anteroposterior X-ray image. (**b**) Routine epidurogram shows no contrast above the level of L5–S1, lateral X-ray image. (**c**) the ventral epidural space epidurogram obtained after hydrostatic (normal saline, 10 cc), mechanical, and chemical (hyaluronidase, 1500 U) adhesiolysis, anteroposterior X-ray image. (**d**) the ventral epidural space epidurogram obtained after hydrostatic (normal saline, 10 cc), mechanical, and chemical (hyaluronidase, 1500 U) adhesiolysis, lateral X-ray image

Step 6 Adhesiolysis Techniques

Check the "scarred in" area with the contrast agent in the real-time image. When contrast medium is injected into the blood vessel, the catheter must be repositioned. In particular, if the contrast medium is being injected into the artery, positioning is absolutely necessary. If intravascular injection is not confirmed, inject 1500 U of hyaluronidase dissolved in 10 mL of physiological saline. Hyaluronidase at normal PH is more effective, and injection is recommended.

Observe for "opening up" (visualization) of the "scarred in" nerve root (Fig. 6.8) [16, 17]. A 3 mL test dose of a 10 mL local anesthetic and steroid solution is then given. If, after five minutes, there is no evidence of intrathecal or intravascular injection of medication, inject the remaining 7 mL of the solution.

Ropivacaine is used instead of bupivacaine for two reasons:

1. Preferential sensory versus a motor block
2. Less cardiotoxic

Step 7 Postoperative Treatment After the Use of a Soft Catheter

Remove the guide needle while confirming with fluoroscopy whether the soft catheter is continuously positioned on the lesion. The soft catheter is fixed to the skin using a non-absorbable suture and attached to the skin through an anvil dressing. Various drugs can be applied to the lesion through a catheter for 3 days. Currently, steroids, local anesthetics, and hyaluronidase are directly injected, and the catheter is removed on the same day.

6.5 Complications

As with all invasive treatments, bleeding, infection, and nerve damage can occur with PEN. PEN is a procedure performed in the epidural space, which may cause cerebrospinal fluid leakage and headaches, and may cause neurological sequelae due to nerve compression caused by injections.

During the PEN procedure, utmost care should be taken not to puncture the dura mater. For this purpose, it is recommended to use fluoroscopy.

In addition, there are retrospective review of 250 patients reporting complications such as bending needle tip (4.8%), amputation of catheter tip (1.2%), catheter remnant (0.4%), and epidural abscess (1.2%) [18]. Another large study reported a high incidence of complications of intravascular injection (11.6%), transient nerve stimulation (1.9%), and dura puncture (1.8%) in 10,000 patients [19].

6.6 Outcomes

PEN has used an important treatment option for patients with intractable cervical, thoracic, and lumbar pain. These studies show that patients experience significant pain relief and restoration of function. Manchikanti et al.'s suggest that the amount and duration of pain relief can be improved by repeat procedures. Several reported studies of failed back surgery and spinal stenosis show 75% and 80% improvement in clinical and functional improvements at 12 months' follow-up, respectively [2–9]. There have been no negative studies to date where the lysis target was the ventrolateral epidural space. Evolution in recognition of the importance of catheters and drug delivery locations, along with the need for physicians to acquire the skills to perform appropriate procedures, can be seen in recent research.

6.7 Keys to Successful Intervention

PEN have multiple steps, including needle position, catheter advance and placement, adhesiolysis, and the injection the medications. All these steps should be accomplished safely and effectively. Catheter routes are planned preoperatively and changed based on real-time imaging during catheter advancement to obtain the correct position. The catheter should be handled gently to avoid injuring the surrounding structures such as dura and root. An epidurogram should be performed before adhesiolysis to confirm that the catheter is positioned correctly. The appropriate use of all three adhesiolysis techniques facilitates epidural scar lysis. At all points during the procedure, the patient's safety is the first concern. If the patient complained intolerable pain or neurological deterioration, the procedure should be stopped immediately.

6.8 Current Limitations

The action mechanism of PEN remains controversial. The evidence that adhesions are related to spinal symptoms is still weak. Some investigators have suggested that hyaluronidase has no benefit in PEN, and it made the anaphylaxis. Hypertonic saline may have serious side effects, although it improves surgical outcomes. Further, the suffix "-plasty," which indicates a surgical procedure, is inappropriate for the minimally invasive EI procedure.

6.9 Future Perspectives

PEN is a minimally invasive treatment method with obvious advantages such as short hospital stay and postoperative epidural scar removal without general anesthesia in an aging society. Numerous studies also support the use of ambulatory PENs for the treatment of FBSS syndrome, spinal stenosis, neuromuscular pain, and axial pain that is refractory to less invasive procedures. Therefore, PEN is an important part of the interventional repertoire for the treatment of low back pain that is refractory to conventional treatments such as ESI.

References

1. Oh CH, Ji GY, Shin DA, Cho PG, Yoon SH. Clinical course of cervical percutaneous epidural neuroplasty in single-level cervical disc disease with 12-month follow-up. Pain Physician. 2017;20:E941–9.
2. Ji GY, Oh CH, Moon B, Choi SH, Shin DA, Yoon YS, et al. Efficacy of percutaneous epidural neuroplasty does not correlate with dural sac cross-sectional area in single level disc disease. Yonsei Med J. 2015;56:691–7.
3. Manchikanti L, Singh V, Cash KA, Pampati V. Assessment of effectiveness of percutaneous adhesiolysis and caudal epidural injections in managing post lumbar surgery syndrome: 2-year follow-up of a randomized, controlled trial. J Pain Res. 2012;5:597–608.
4. Manchikanti L, Singh V, Cash KA, Pampati V, Datta S. A comparative effectiveness evaluation of percutaneous adhesiolysis and epidural steroid injections in managing lumbar post surgery syndrome: a ran-

domized equivalence controlled trial. Pain Physician. 2009;12:E355–68.

5. Heavner JE, Racz GB, Raj P. Percutaneous epidural neuroplasty: prospective evaluation of 0.9% NaCl versus 10% NaCl with or without hyaluronidase. Reg Anesth Pain Med. 1999;24:202–7.
6. Manchikanti L, Rivera JJ, Pampati V, Damron KS, McManus CD, Brandon DE, et al. One day lumbar epidural adhesiolysis and hypertonic saline neurolysis in treatment of chronic low back pain: a randomized, double-blind trial. Pain Physician. 2004;7:177–86.
7. Veihelmann A, Devens C, Trouillier H, Birkenmaier C, Gerdesmeyer L, Refior HJ. Epidural neuroplasty versus physiotherapy to relieve pain in patients with sciatica: a prospective randomized blinded clinical trial. J Orthop Sci. 2006;11:365–9.
8. Manchikanti L, Falco FJ, Singh V, Pampati V, Parr AT, Benyamin RM, et al. Utilization of interventional techniques in managing chronic pain in the Medicare population: analysis of growth patterns from 2000 to 2011. Pain Physician. 2012;(115):E969–82.
9. Park CH, Lee SH, Jung JY. Dural sac cross-sectional area does not correlate with efficacy of percutaneous adhesiolysis in single level lumbar spinal stenosis. Pain Physician. 2011;14:377–82.
10. Racz G. Techniques of neurolysis. Boston: Kluwer Academic Publishers; 1989. p. 218.
11. Lee N, Ji GY, Yi S, do Yoon H, Shin DA, Kim KN, et al. Finite element analysis of the effect of epidural adhesions. Pain Physician. 2016;19:E787–93.
12. Manchikanti L, Abdi S, Atluri S, Benyamin RM, Boswell MV, Buenaventura RM, et al. An update of comprehensive evidence-based guidelines for interventional techniques in chronic spinal pain. Part II: guidance and recommendations. Pain Physician. 2013;16(2 Suppl):S49–283.
13. Cooper RG, Freemont AJ, Hoyland JA, Jenkins JP, West CG, Illingworth KJ, et al. Herniated intervertebral disc-associated periradicular fibrosis and vascular abnormalities occur without inflammatory cell infiltration. Spine (Phila Pa 1976). 1995;20:591–8.
14. McCarron RF, Wimpee MW, Hudkins PG, Laros GS. The inflammatory effect of nucleus pulposus. A possible element in the pathogenesis of low-back pain. Spine (Phila Pa 1976). 1987;12:760–4.
15. Manchikanti L, Falco FJE, Singh V, Benyamin RM, Racz GB, Helm S 2nd, et al. An update of comprehensive evidence-based guidelines for interventional techniques in chronic spinal pain. Part I: introduction and general considerations. Pain Physician. 2013;16(2 Suppl):S1–48.
16. Park SH, Ji GY, Cho PG, Shin DA, Yoon YS, Kim KN, et al. Clinical significance of epidurography contrast patterns after adhesiolysis during lumbar percutaneous epidural neuroplasty. Pain Res Manag. 2018;2018:6268045–8.
17. Moon BJ, Yi S, Ha Y, Kim KN, Yoon DH, Shin DA. Clinical efficacy and safety of trans-sacral epiduroscopic laser decompression compared to percutaneous epidural neuroplasty. Pain Res Manag. 2019;2019:2893460.
18. Talu GK, Erdine S. Complications of epidural neuroplasty: a retrospective evaluation. Neuromodulation. 2003;6:237–47.
19. Park Y, Lee WY, Ahn JK, Nam HS, Lee KH. Percutaneous adhesiolysis versus transforaminal epidural steroid injection for the treatment of chronic radicular pain caused by lumbar foraminal spinal stenosis: a retrospective comparative study. Ann Rehabil Med. 2015;39:941–9.

7 Balloon Neuroplasty Using an Inflatable Balloon (ZiNeu) Catheter: A Technical Note

Seong-Soo Choi and Doo-Hwan Kim

7.1 Introduction

The populace of Korea has become an aged society, defined as one in which more than 14% of the population is ≥65 years old [1, 2]. The incidence of spinal diseases has increased as the population aged. In patients over 60 years of age with a spinal disease, spinal stenosis is the most frequent diagnosis and accounts for the largest proportion of total medical costs [1]. Although treatment modalities for spinal stenosis vary, the therapeutic effect of conservative treatment is limited in some cases [3]. PEN has been widely used in cases where conventional treatment has failed (e.g., ESI for chronic spinal stenosis) [4, 5]. The newly introduced combined epidural adhesiolysis and balloon decompression using an inflatable balloon catheter (balloon neuroplasty) has resulted in excellent clinical outcomes in patients with chronic refractory spinal stenosis [6–8]. Here, we provide a physician's guide to balloon neuroplasty that describes the procedure techniques to enhance the reader's understanding of this intervention and facilitate skillful use of the catheter to maximize the clinical effect.

PEN, often called epidural adhesiolysis, was first introduced by Racz as a treatment for chronic LBP, with or without radiating leg pain, caused by epidural adhesions after lumbar spine surgery [9]. PEN frees up nerves and breaks down scar tissue through mechanical or chemical action, thereby reducing perineural inflammation and edema by effectively delivering corticosteroids and local anesthetics to specific target lesions. Based on these mechanism, PEN can reduce pain and other neurological symptoms [9]. PEN has been performed using a shear-resistant catheter (the Racz-type) or a more steerable navigation catheter (NaviCath, Myelotec, Roswell, GA, USA) traditionally [10, 11]. Recently, PEN has been widely used in patients with spinal stenosis, a disc herniation, or post-spinal surgery syndrome, which can lead to chronic LBP or leg pain secondary to epidural adhesions. The effectiveness of PEN for the treatment of chronic refractory symptoms that persist after conventional treatment such as ESI is relatively well established [12]. However, the long-term effects (i.e., over 6 months) of conventional epidural neuroplasty are uncertain and controversial [13].

Previous report indicates that transforaminal balloon treatment improves functional capacity and reduces LBP and leg pain in patients with refractory spinal stenosis [14]. Based on this research, the Zigzag-motion Inflatable Neuroplasty (ZiNeu) catheter with an inflatable balloon (JUVENUI, Seongnam, Korea) was introduced for the treatment of epidural adhesiolysis (Fig. 7.1) [15]. PEN, using a balloon-inflatable catheter that can perform combined

S.-S. Choi (✉) · D.-H. Kim
Department of Anesthesiology and Pain Medicine, Asan Medical Center, Seoul, Republic of Korea
e-mail: choiss@amc.seoul.kr; dh_kim@amc.seoul.kr

S.-H. Lee (ed.), *Minimally Invasive Spine Interventions*,
https://doi.org/10.1007/978-981-16-9547-6_7

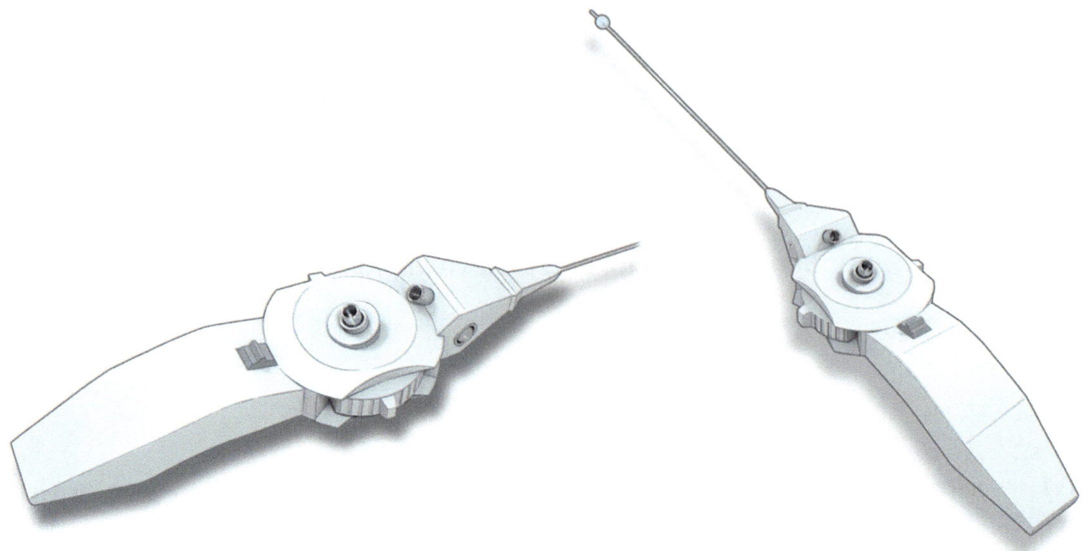

Fig. 7.1 Zigzag-motion Inflatable Neuroplasty (ZiNeu) catheter with an inflatable balloon

epidural adhesiolysis and balloon decompression (balloon neuroplasty), yielded significant pain relief and functional improvement in patients with central or foraminal spinal stenosis up to 12 months after the procedure [6, 16]. Balloon neuroplasty also produced successful clinical outcomes in patients with failed back surgery syndrome (FBSS) [17, 18] and seemed to be superior to PEN using a conventional non-balloon catheter, such as the Racz catheter for central spinal stenosis with neurogenic claudication [19]. Furthermore, balloon neuroplasty was effective in patients with intractable lumbar spinal stenosis who were unresponsive to previous conventional PEN [7]. These results indicate that balloon neuroplasty can be an effective alternative to conventional PEN.

PEN produces good clinical outcomes in patients with chronic back pain and epidural adhesions. However, a poor clinical effect after PEN is not uncommon and is associated with incomplete adhesiolysis due to technical difficulties or severe or multiple adhesions [4, 11]. Correct placement of the balloon-inflatable catheter at the target lesion and skillful manipulation of the instrument (e.g., rotation, bending, and inflation and deflation of the balloon) are especially necessary for good long-term effects after balloon neuroplasty [8]. However, there is no clear and detailed technical description of balloon neuroplasty. Here, we provide a technical guide to facilitate the accurate and skillful performance of balloon neuroplasty and maximize the clinical effects of this procedure.

7.2 Indications and Contraindications

The studies performed to identify factors that predict a successful outcome after balloon neuroplasty [6–8, 16, 18–20] demonstrate that the ideal indications are as follows:

1. Lumbar central or foraminal stenosis with chronic radicular pain and intermittent neurogenic claudication but no back pain.
2. Refractory symptoms; the improvement is less than one month after an epidural block or conventional PEN.
3. Symptomatic pathological lesions including degenerative IVDs that cause chronic perineural adhesions or substantially contribute to stenosis.
4. Mild to moderate stenosis.

Patients with a neuropathic component (e.g., diabetic neuropathy) and co-existing lower back pain may experience a poor outcome after balloon neuroplasty [6]. In patients with FBSS, early intervention with balloon neuroplasty may be associated with a favorable outcome, although it has limited effectiveness [18]. Therefore, balloon neuroplasty should be carefully considered in this population. Additionally, contrast medium distribution over the entire target area may be needed, and if multiple targets are present, more than 50% should be successfully ballooned to achieve a positive clinical outcome [8, 21]. Factors that predict a favorable outcome after balloon neuroplasty are summarized in Table 7.1.

The contraindications to balloon neuroplasty are similar to those of conventional PEN and include:

1. Patient refusal.
2. Progressive neurological deficits or motor weakness.
3. Coagulopathy.
4. Signs of infection.
5. Pregnancy or nursing.
6. Allergy to local anesthetics, steroids, or contrast agents.
7. Unstable medical or psychiatric condition.

Table 7.1 Predictive factors of a favorable outcome after balloon neuroplasty

1. Pathology
– Perineural adhesion secondary to chronic degenerative disc disease (herniated intervertebral disc)
– Lumbar spinal stenosis mainly caused by degenerative disc
– Mild to moderate stenosis
2. Related symptoms
– Chronic radicular pain without lower back pain (neurogenic claudication)
– Minimal neuropathic component (e.g., diabetic neuropathy)
– Less than 14 months of pain duration after lumbar surgery
3. Procedural elements
– More than 50% of multiple target sites ballooned
– Complete contrast dye spread after ballooning

7.3 Methods

7.3.1 ZiNeu Catheter: Caudal Approach

Step 1 Patient Preparation
The intervention is conducted with the patient in the prone position on an operating table with a slightly high pillow beneath the abdomen to minimize lumbar lordosis. This position can lower resistance to catheter insertion because the spinal canal becomes relatively straight. A povidone-iodine solution is used for skin disinfection. Before disinfecting the operative site, a small gauze pad should be placed in the area between the coccyx and anus to prevent the solution from flowing into the anus.

Step 2 ZiNeu Catheter Preparation
A 10-ml syringe filled with approximately 3–4 ml of contrast medium is connected to the contrast inlet of the ZiNeu catheter to remove air from the catheter and inject contrast medium. The syringe plunger is pulled sufficiently to maintain strong negative pressure for 2–3 s. The plunger is then released (Fig. 7.2). This maneuver removes the air from the catheter and fills the space with the contrast medium. Then, a 1-ml Luer-Lock syringe (BD Medical, Franklin Lakes, NJ, USA) containing 0.13 ml of contrast medium is connected to the contrast inlet of the ZiNeu catheter for ballooning (Fig. 7.3).

Step 3 Local Anesthesia and Approach
After local infiltration of 1% lidocaine sufficient for anesthesia, a 10-gauge epidural guide needle (or sheath with stylet) is inserted into the caudal epidural space through the sacral hiatus under fluoroscopic guidance. When inserting the epidural guide needle into the skin, it should be advanced with its bevel facing upward. When the needle tip passes through the sacrococcygeal ligament, the needle should be immediately rotated by 180° (bevel facing downward) to minimize damage to the sacrum from the needle tip. Subsequently, the needle is advanced further by 1–3 cm. Then, the guide needle stylet is removed, and the guide sheath is retained.

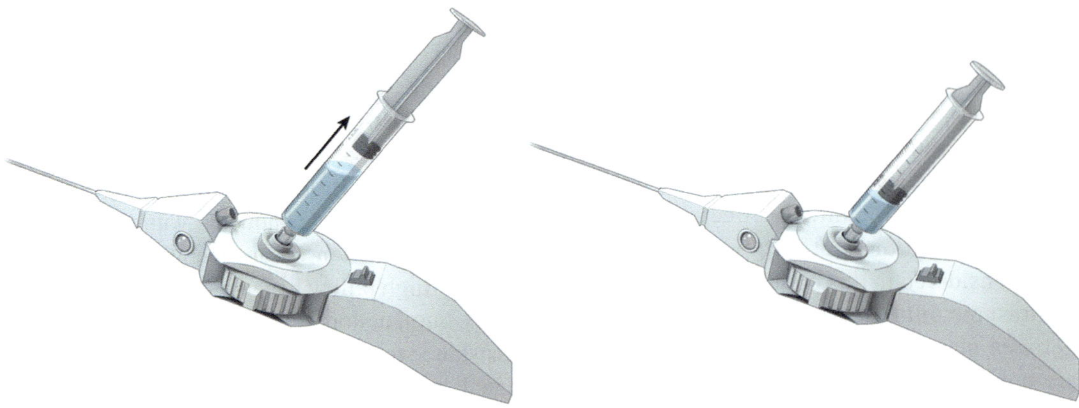

Fig. 7.2 The syringe plunger of ZiNeu catheter for removing air from the catheter

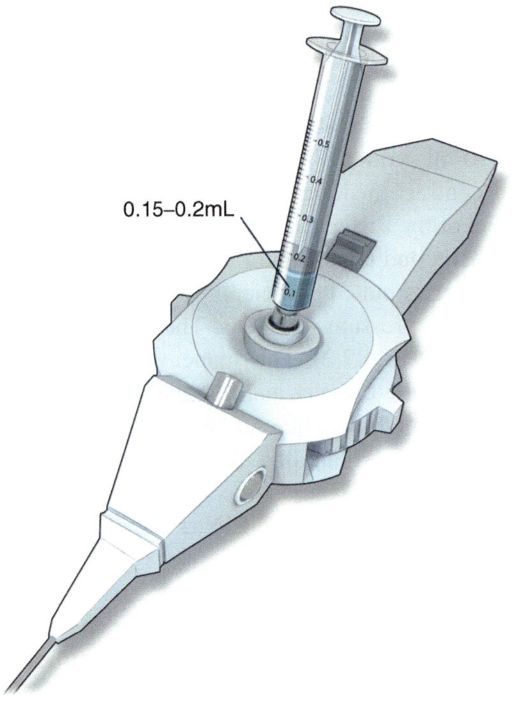

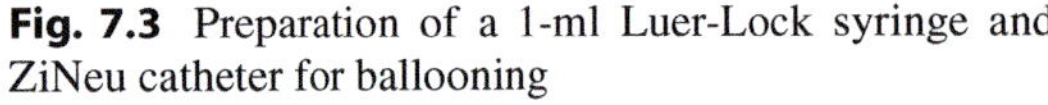

Fig. 7.3 Preparation of a 1-ml Luer-Lock syringe and ZiNeu catheter for ballooning

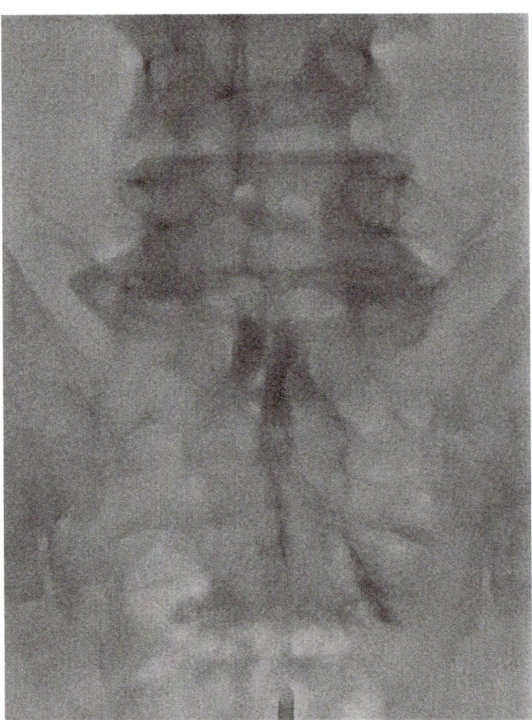

Fig. 7.4 Obtaining epidurogram before the balloon neuroplasty

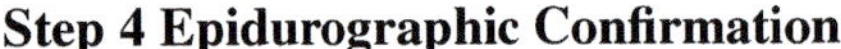

Step 4 Epidurographic Confirmation

The contrast medium is administered to identify the epidural space. The guide needle should be immediately repositioned if intravascular or subarachnoid contrast dispersion occurs. After confirming proper guide needle position in the epidural space, an epidurogram is obtained to assess the stenotic region in the epidural space and the filling defect using approximately 5–8 mL of a solution of contrast diluted with 1% lidocaine (Fig. 7.4). Hyaluronidase can be added to the solution in this step. Performing an epidurogram in this way provides regional anesthesia adequate to increase the procedure success rate by reducing procedural pain. However, care should be taken to avoid injecting the mixture into the intrathecal space.

Step 5 Insertion of the Catheter and Targeting

After verifying the target area, the ZiNeu catheter is advanced through the guide needle to the target lesion. This step is accomplished by catheter manipulation, including advancement, withdrawal, rotation, and occasional bending of the catheter tip. It is especially important to bend the catheter tip slightly and rotate the catheter body delicately to reach the target site easily and accurately. The ZiNeu catheter balloon neuroplasty should be conducted gently at appropriate target sites determined by the epidurogram, lesion location on the lumbar MRI, and symptomatology. The anterior and posterior epidural spaces, the lateral recess area, and each intervertebral foramen are the main target sites.

Step 6 Epidural Adhesiolysis and Balloon Decompression

Combined epidural adhesiolysis and balloon decompression are performed using a gentle side-to-side movement of the catheter with intermittent ballooning (Fig. 7.5). An inflatable balloon is attached to the end of the catheter tip. The balloon is filled with 0.13 mL of contrast agent using a 1-mL Luer-Lock syringe, and the ballooning maneuver lasts a maximum of 5 s. More importantly, the balloon should be inflated slowly and gently while observing the patient's response. Ballooning should be done only to the extent that the patient can tolerate it, and it is not necessary to inflate the balloon maximally. The extent of balloon inflation should be limited to prevent ischemic nerve damage if the patient complains of moderate to severe pain. The

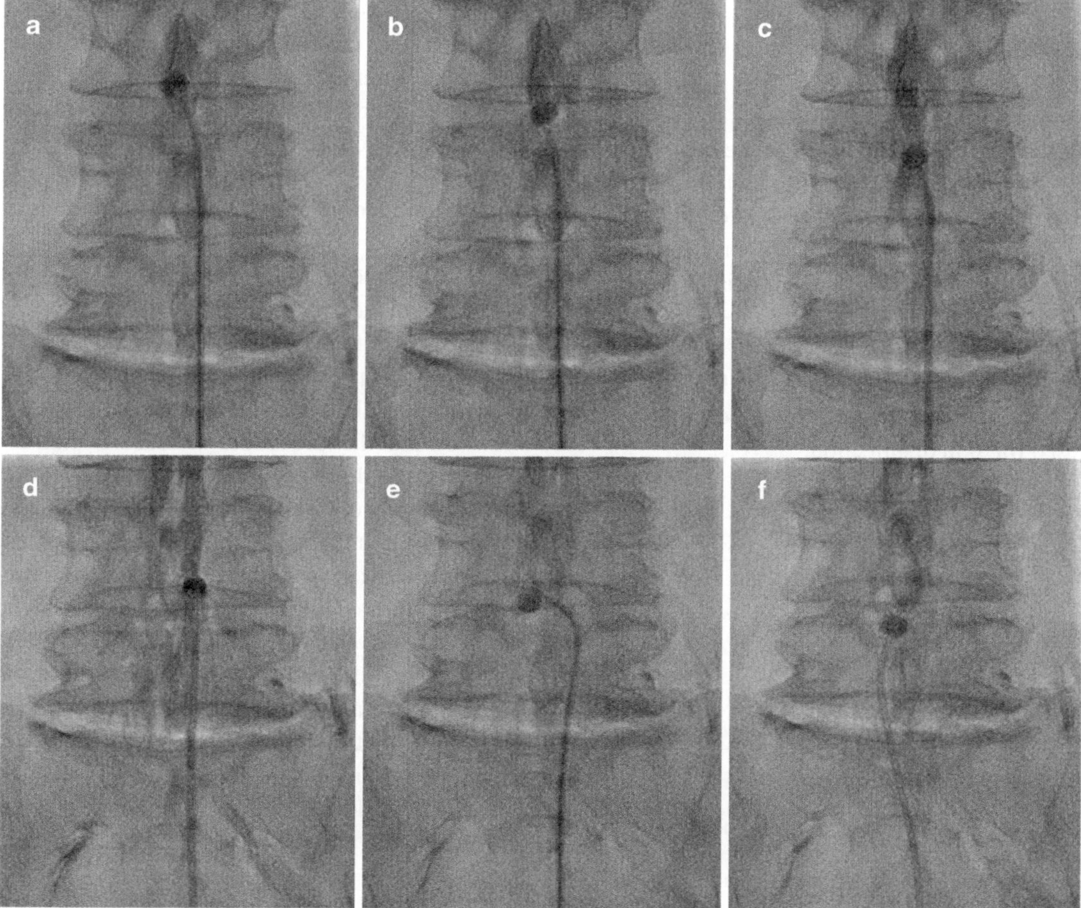

Fig. 7.5 Combined epidural adhesiolysis and balloon decompression using a gentle side-to-side movement of the catheter with ballooning for central spinal lesion

catheter is moved only when the balloon is deflated. The balloon is repeatedly inflated and deflated throughout the target region. After epidural adhesiolysis and balloon decompression, 1 mL of undiluted contrast is used to exclude subarachnoid or intravascular injection and ensure the reduction of the previously identified filling defects. Then, 2 mL of 1% lidocaine with 5 mg of dexamethasone is administered at each target site.

7.3.2 Zineu-F Catheter: Transforaminal Approach

Although this catheter is thin (approximately 2 Fr), it is strengthened by a reinforcing guidewire (Fig. 7.6). It is simple to operate and useful for approaching pathological stenotic lesions, resulting in more than moderate foraminal stenosis. Therefore, it is suitable for a transforaminal approach.

Step 1 Patient Preparation
The patient is placed in the prone position with a high pillow underneath the abdomen to reduce lumbar lordosis. The success rate of procedures performed on the L5 intervertebral foramen can be increased by reducing lordosis to prevent the L5 intervertebral foramen from being obscured by the iliac crest. Therefore, this procedure requires a higher pillow than that needed for the caudal approach. A povidone-iodine solution is used for skin disinfection.

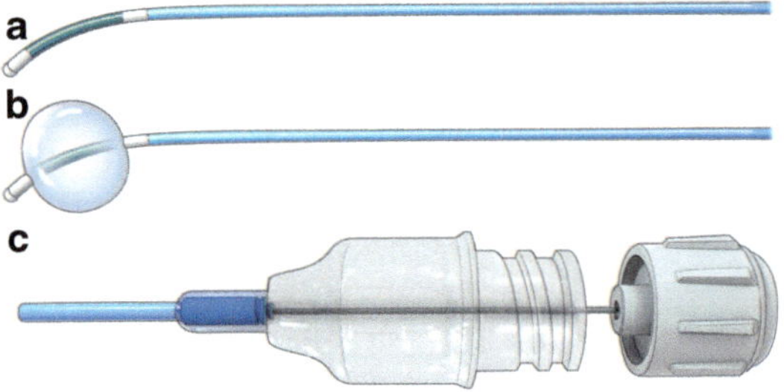

Fig. 7.6 Zineu-F catheter for transforaminal approach. (**a**) Deflated state. (**b**) Inflated state. (**c**) Reinforcing guidewire pre-inserted into the catheter

Step 2 Preparation of the ZiNeu-F Catheter
A guidewire is already inside the ZiNeu-F catheter. Unlike the caudal approach using the ZiNeu catheter, this procedure requires catheter air replacement with contrast medium after the catheter reaches the target area and just before the balloon decompression.

Step 3 Local Anesthesia and Approach
After sterile preparation, the skin and soft tissue are anesthetized with 1% lidocaine. Either a guide needle or a sheath can be used. The use of a guide sheath can lower the risk of balloon rupture. The target intervertebral foramen is determined by clinical symptoms or the pathological lesion on lumbar MRI. In the oblique view with an angle of 30–35°, the insertion point is the inferolateral area of the intervertebral foramen. If the foramen (particularly targeting the L5–S1 foramen) is obscured in the 30° oblique view due to a high iliac crest, a contralateral interlaminar retrograde foraminal approach rather than transforaminal approach is considered for ZiNeu-F catheter insertion [22].

Step 4 Epidurographic Confirmation and Targeting
The guide needle should be inserted along the nerve root in the safe triangle in the superomedial direction and then advanced to the 6 o'clock position of the pedicle in the oblique fluoroscopic view. The needle tip should be checked in the AP view during the procedure to ensure that the guide needle does not pass the midline of the pedicle to prevent a dura puncture. If the needle tip passes through the anterior epidural space and reaches the posterior surface of the vertebral body, a pre-procedural epidurogram should be obtained and the needle retracted by about 2–3 mm to allow catheter advancement into the anterior epidural space and prevent balloon catheter tearing on the sharp edge of the needle bevel. The needle tip is held outside the foraminal inlet. Then, the ZiNeu-F catheter, with its enclosed guidewire, is advanced slightly to the target foramen.

Step 5 Epidural Adhesiolysis and Balloon Decompression

When the ZiNeu-F catheter reaches the target area, the guidewire is removed, and the air inside the catheter is replaced with the contrast medium. A 5-ml syringe filled with approximately 2 ml of contrast medium is connected to the catheter. The plunger is forcefully pulled back and released to expel the air inside the balloon catheter, and the contrast medium automatically flows into the catheter (Fig. 7.7). Then, a 1-ml Luer-Lock syringe containing 0.1 ml of a contrast medium is connected to the catheter for ballooning (Fig. 7.8). Initially, only 0.05 ml of contrast medium should be slowly introduced into the catheter. Then, careful mechanical adhesiolysis is conducted by repeatedly inflating and deflating the balloon throughout the entire target area under fluoroscopy. The target usually includes 3 to 5 consecutive points between the lateral recess and the outlet of the intervertebral foramen (Fig. 7.9). Importantly, the balloon should be inflated slowly and gradually for no more than 5 s at a time while observing the patient's response. The balloon is usually inflated three times at each point between the lateral recess and the outlet of the intervertebral foramen. After the last deflation, the catheter is withdrawn. The catheter should only be moved when the balloon is deflated. After performing

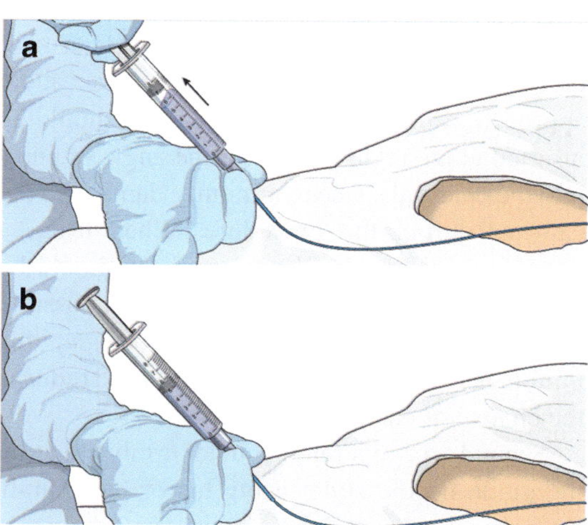

Fig. 7.7 Air-expelling and contrast filling

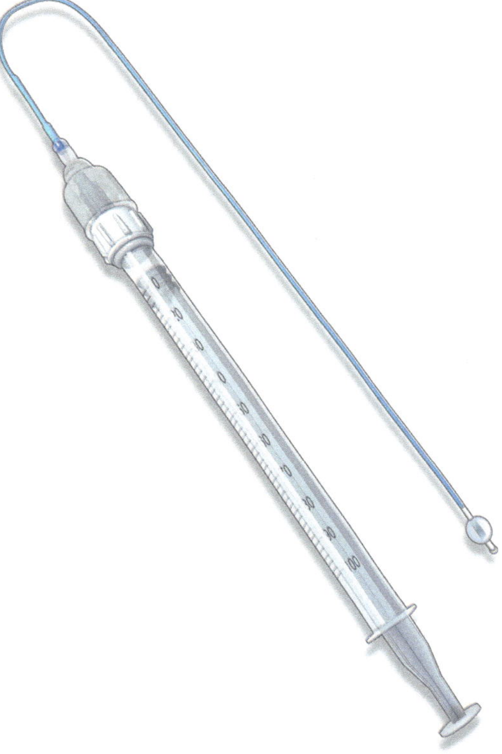

Fig. 7.8 Preparation of a 1-ml Luer-Lock syringe and Zineu-F catheter for transforaminal ballooning

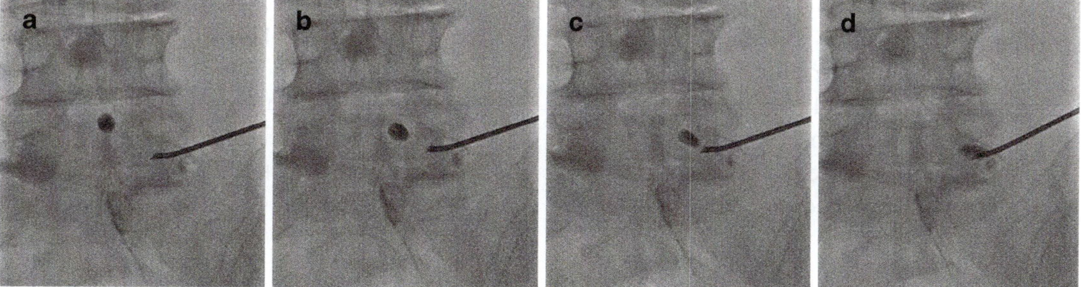

Fig. 7.9 Technique for stepwise transforaminal balloon neuroplasty

the first balloon decompression with a small amount of contrast, the catheter is reinserted, and the second balloon decompression is conducted with up to 0.3 mL of contrast medium.

Step 6 Injection and Post-epidurogram
The extent of balloon inflation is adjusted to the degree of procedural pain; if moderate to severe pain occurs during balloon inflation, the operator should stop inflating the balloon. In the second round of inflation and deflation, the patient will tolerate a greater degree of inflation because the elasticity of the balloon is increased, and the perineural space is expanded. After completing balloon decompression and adhesiolysis, the guide needle is reinserted for an ESI. A post-procedure epidurogram is obtained to assess the degree of filling defect improvement. Then, 3 mL of a mixture of 1% lidocaine, 5 mg of dexamethasone, and 1500 IU of hyaluronidase is administered.

7.4 Procedure-Related Precautions

7.4.1 Methods for Preventing Balloon Rupture

Using an unbreakable balloon could be dangerous because it could exert excessive pressure on the surrounding nerves, resulting in ischemic damage. Therefore, a balloon that ruptures under excessive pressure is very important for patient safety. Nevertheless, a balloon rupture before the completion of the procedure could be problematic. Therefore, we recommend several precautions to ensure safe balloon inflation and avoid balloon rupture during the procedure.

First, a guide sheath should be used instead of a guide needle, especially by novices. Microdamage to the balloon surface can often occur when the balloon catheter tip passes through the guide needle, which could increase the likelihood of balloon rupture during the procedure.

Second, when inflating the balloon, the contrast medium should be injected slowly and gently to minimize the risk of rupture. Rapid injection of the contrast agent during balloon inflation can cause high pressure within the balloon, leading to balloon rupture and severe pain.

Third, it is essential to inflate the balloon in a gradual, stepwise manner; only 0.05 ml of contrast medium should be injected during the first inflation and 0.1 ml of contrast medium during the second and third inflations. This practice increases the elasticity of the balloon and expands the stenotic region while lowering the risk of balloon rupture due to high pressure, thus resulting in less procedural pain.

7.4.2 Methods for Preventing Catheter Damage

Although a rare occurrence, the guide needle can damage the catheter. Several methods can help prevent this event. First, when using a caudal approach, if possible, the guide needle should be inserted at an angle parallel to the angle of entry into the epidural space to minimize damage to the catheter during the procedure. When using a transforaminal approach, the catheter should be inserted by moving it down as far as possible toward the intervertebral foraminal angle; this minimizes resistance during insertion and reduces the chance of catheter damage.

Second, the operator should firmly position the guide needle stylet using his or her thumb. Stylet displacement during insertion of the guide needle can cause guide needle tip damage. Balloon catheter movement through the damaged guide needle can also lead to balloon or catheter damage. Additionally, when the catheter is withdrawn, it should be pulled slowly. If any resistance is detected, the bevel of the needle should be slightly rotated until the operator finds the specific angle at which it can be withdrawn without resistance. If the catheter cannot be withdrawn despite various maneuvers, the guide needle and catheter should be removed together.

7.4.3 Perioperative Complications and Management

Although relatively rare, perioperative complications can occur after balloon neuroplasty. According to previous reports [8, 21], a dural puncture was found in 3.3–3.9% of patients, and subdural injection was suspected in 1.9%. If a dural puncture or subdural injection is suspected during balloon neuroplasty, the procedure should be stopped immediately. Additionally, the incidence of vascular injection was 1.5%, and 1.9% of patients experienced hypotension during balloon neuroplasty [8, 21]. However, none of the patients with a complication had persistent neurologic deficits, and all were discharged after a short period of bed rest. The most common complication may be post-procedural pain. Therefore, the patient should be informed that pain or discomfort can persist for 2–3 days after balloon decompression.

Although almost all post-procedural pain subsides within the first several days, in rare cases, the patient may experience severe or persistent pain for over 10 days. Therefore, post-procedural pain should be managed carefully, and in such cases, an epidural block using a local anesthetic alone could reduce the pain.

7.5 Conclusions

Balloon neuroplasty can lead to significant pain relief and functional improvement in patients with chronic refractory pain associated with lumbar spinal stenosis and could be a useful alternative to overcome the limitations of conventional epidural neuroplasty. Because an accurately and skillfully executed balloon neuroplasty can provide a good, long-term clinical effect, it is essential to understand the features of the ZiNeu catheter and learn to manipulate it successfully when performing balloon decompression. Therefore, this technical guide may be of value to physicians who conduct balloon neuroplasty with the ZiNeu catheter.

References

1. Lee CH, Chung CK, Kim CH, Kwon JW. Health care burden of spinal diseases in the Republic of Korea: analysis of a nationwide database from 2012 through 2016. Neurospine. 2018;15:66–76.
2. Tahara Y. Cardiopulmonary resuscitation in a super-aging society- is there an age limit for cardiopulmonary resuscitation? Circ J. 2016;80:1102–3.
3. Jamison DE, Hsu E, Cohen SP. Epidural adhesiolysis: an evidence-based review. J Neurosurg Sci. 2014;58:65–76.
4. Hsu E, Atanelov L, Plunkett AR, Chai N, Chen Y, Cohen SP. Epidural lysis of adhesions for failed back surgery and spinal stenosis: factors associated with treatment outcome. Anesth Analg. 2014;118:215–24.
5. Lee F, Jamison DE, Hurley RW, Cohen SP. Epidural lysis of adhesions. Korean J Pain. 2014;27:3–15.
6. Choi SS, Lee JH, Kim D, Kim HK, Lee S, Song KJ, et al. Effectiveness and factors associated with epidural decompression and adhesiolysis using a balloon-inflatable catheter in chronic lumbar spinal stenosis: 1-year follow-up. Pain Med. 2016;17:476–87.
7. Karm MH, Yoon SH, Seo DK, Lee S, Lee Y, Cho SS, et al. Combined epidural adhesiolysis and balloon decompression can be effective in intractable lumbar spinal stenosis patients unresponsive to previous epidural adhesiolysis. Medicine. 2019;98:e15114.
8. Park JY, Ji GY, Lee SW, Park JK, Ha D, Park Y, et al. Relationship of success rate for balloon adhesiolysis with clinical outcomes in chronic intractable lumbar radicular pain: a multicenter prospective study. J Clin Med. 2019;8:606.
9. Racz GB, Holubec JT. Lysis of adhesions in the epidural space. In: Racz GB, editor. Techniques of neurolysis. Boston: Kluwer Academic; 1989.
10. Racz GB, Heavner JE, Trescot A. Percutaneous lysis of epidural adhesions--evidence for safety and efficacy. Pain Pract. 2008;8:277–86.
11. Lee JH, Lee SH. Clinical effectiveness of percutaneous adhesiolysis and predictive factors of treatment efficacy in patients with lumbosacral spinal stenosis. Pain Med. 2013;14:1497–504.
12. Kim HJ, Rim BC, Lim JW, Park NK, Kang TW, Sohn MK, et al. Efficacy of epidural neuroplasty versus transforaminal epidural steroid injection for the radiating pain caused by a herniated lumbar disc. Ann Rehabil Med. 2013;37:824–31.
13. Manchikanti L, Abdi S, Atluri S, Benyamin RM, Boswell MV, Buenaventura RM, et al. An update of comprehensive evidence-based guidelines for interventional techniques in chronic spinal pain. Part II: guidance and recommendations. Pain Physician. 2013;16:S49–283.
14. Kim SH, Choi WJ, Suh JH, Jeon SR, Hwang CJ, Koh WU, et al. Effects of transforaminal balloon treatment in patients with lumbar foraminal stenosis:

a randomized, controlled, double-blind trial. Pain Physician. 2013;16:213–24.

15. Choi SS, Joo EY, Hwang BS, Lee JH, Lee G, Suh JH, et al. A novel balloon-inflatable catheter for percutaneous epidural adhesiolysis and decompression. Korean J Pain. 2014;27:178–85.
16. Kim DH, Cho SS, Moon YJ, Kwon K, Lee K, Leem JG, et al. Factors associated with successful responses to transforaminal balloon adhesiolysis for chronic lumbar foraminal stenosis: retrospective study. Pain Physician. 2017;20:E841–8.
17. Hwang BY, Ko HS, Suh JH, Shin JW, Leem JG, Lee JD. Clinical experiences of performing transforaminal balloon adhesiolysis in patients with failed back surgery syndrome: two cases report. Korean J Anesthesiol. 2014;66:169–72.
18. Oh Y, Shin DA, Kim DJ, Cho W, Na T, Leem JG, et al. Effectiveness of and factors associated with balloon adhesiolysis in patients with lumbar postlaminectomy syndrome: a retrospective study. J Clin Med. 2020;9:1144.
19. Karm MH, Choi SS, Kim DH, Park JY, Lee S, Park JK, et al. Percutaneous epidural adhesiolysis using inflatable balloon catheter and balloon-less catheter in central lumbar spinal stenosis with neurogenic claudication: a randomized controlled trial. Pain Physician. 2018;21:593–606.
20. Oh Y, Kim DH, Park JY, Ji GY, Shin DA, Lee SW, et al. Factors associated with successful response to balloon decompressive adhesiolysis neuroplasty in patients with chronic lumbar foraminal stenosis. J Clin Med. 2019;8:1766.
21. Kim DH, Ji GY, Kwon HJ, Na T, Shin JW, Shin DA, et al. Contrast dispersion on epidurography may be associated with clinical outcomes after percutaneous epidural neuroplasty using an inflatable balloon catheter. Pain Med. 2020;21:677–85.
22. Kim CS, Moon YJ, Kim JW, Hyun DM, Son SL, Shin JW, et al. Transforaminal epidural balloon adhesiolysis via a contralateral retrograde interlaminar approach: a retrospective analysis and technical considerations. J Clin Med. 2020;9:981.

8 Percutaneous Discoplasty: Nucleoplasty and Annuloplasty

Sang-Heon Lee, Nackhwan Kim, Richard Derby, and You Ha Kwon

8.1 Introduction

Disc herniation is a common source of acute and chronic radicular pain [1]. Percutaneous decompression techniques include arthroscopic manual extraction and nuclear ablation using plasma or laser-generated heat. Interventionalists typically consider percutaneous techniques for contained disc herniation that ideally have high water content [2]. More recent navigable decompression devices now allow targeted decompression to include noncontained herniated discs [3].

Over 10 years ago, ArthroCare Corporation, Austin, TX, USA, introduced a plasma-generating ablation device, Perc-D SpineWand, to allow percutaneous decompression of the intervertebral disc nucleus. The device uses a straight catheter, and thus, one cannot easily manipulate the tip into central and paracentral lumbar disc herniations.

Based on his clinical experience, Kambin reported that herniation laterality and size are not prognostic outcome indicators. Partial decompression of contained fragments is possible with precise manipulation of an epidural catheter [4]. However, access to extruded and sequestrated fragments was most often impossible [5–7]. To facilitate manipulation within the disc and epidural space, the L'DISQ developed by authors and U & I Corporation, Uijeongbu-si, Gyeonggi-do, Korea, uses a navigable catheter. Preliminary study results by the author showed its efficacy and safety for the treatment of leg pain [3].

Both the SpineWand and L'DISQ devices are used to treat contained disc herniations causing radicular pain, ideally when discography demonstrates concordant pain provocation at low volume and pressure, and the CT-discogram scan documents a small to moderate-sized contained herniation preferably with a wide-neck radial annular tear. Although recent studies by Sim et al. [8] and Bokov et al. reported favorable outcomes postdecompression in patients with extruded discs [9, 10], large extrusions, sequestration, and large herniations more than one-third of the sagittal diameter of the spinal canal are relative contraindications for devices that cannot directly decompress the disc herniation [11].

The rationale for central nuclear decompression attributes efficacy to lowering intradiscal pressure, potentially lowering nerve root pressure by a contained and contiguous herniation. The rationale conceives the disc as a closed hydraulic

S.-H. Lee (✉) · Y. H. Kwon
Department of Spine and Pain Center, Korea University Anam Hospital, Seoul, Republic of Korea

N. Kim
Department of Physical Medicine and Rehabilitation, Korea University Anam Hospital, Seoul, Republic of Korea

R. Derby
Spinal Diagnostics and Treatment Center, Daly City, CA, USA

S.-H. Lee (ed.), *Minimally Invasive Spine Interventions*,
https://doi.org/10.1007/978-981-16-9547-6_8

system where conceptually, a partial decompression of one part of the disc will induce decompression of the entire disc [12]. However, no studies have validated this concept by correlating outcomes with pre- and post-procedural intradiscal pressures.

The evidence that the removal of small volume nuclear tissue leads to significant decreases in intradiscal pressure has been demonstrated in the experiment of bovine disc laser ablation [13]. In addition, modulation of inflammatory cytokines produced by dead and dying nuclear cells could potentially decrease both axial and radicular pain [14, 15].

In this chapter, we review the progress of other minimally invasive spinal intervention techniques and discuss the L'DISQ developers' perspectives on the invention and their plans for this innovative instrument.

8.2 Indications

Indications

- Radicular leg pain caused by a herniated nucleus pulposus.
- MRI evidence of a contained disc herniation, including extrusion.
- Refractory pain after more than 3 months of conservative management.

Contraindications

- Chronic discogenic pain with diffuse circumferential spread of contrast in discography (relative).[1]
- Severe disc degeneration with an intervertebral space less than half heights of adjacent normal disc space or severe deformation of the endplates.
- Disc sequestration.
- Moderate to severe central spinal stenosis.
- Conjoined myelopathy on MRI or any signs of upper motor neuron lesion in case of the cervical HNP.
- Unstable hemodynamic status.
- Spinal malignancy, infection, or bone fracture.

[1] Outcome data needed.

8.3 Central Nuclear Decompression in Contained Disc

A contained disc has an intact outer annulus and will not leak injected nuclear contrast into the epidural space during discography [16].

The use of MRI alone to identify contained versus noncontained herniations has sensitivity, specificity, and accuracy of 72%, 68%, and 70%, respectively [17]. The MRI signs include a base that is less than the distance from the base to the edge of the herniation in the same plane, and an epidurally displaced disc material is continuous with the disc material within the disc space. The craniocaudal length of the base does not exceed the height of the intervertebral space. In contrast, an extruded disc, even if under the peridural membrane or posterior longitudinal ligament, has a noncontiguous disc material extending further into the epidural canal than the base.

Even in weight-bearing extension and in a stenotic canal, the measured epidural pressure is about six times lower than the intradiscal pressures in a disc with an intact annulus [18–20]. Thus, the pressure vector is almost always outward toward the outer annulus and longitudinal ligaments, and although not validated, it is implausible that an extruded disc will decompress into the disc.

8.4 Targeted Decompression Contained and Noncontained HNP

Conceptually, a more robust method of disc decompression is vaporization of the herniated disc rather than the central disc nucleus. By ablating the herniation, one vaporizes the source of inflammation and potentially relieves pressure on the outer annulus, longitudinal ligament, and nerve root [2]. The tradeoff is an increased risk of inadvertent damage to adjacent neurovascular and skeletal structures. Plasma-generating tissue ablation and proportional catheter navigation techniques are crucial to prevent complications (Figs. 8.1 and 8.2). One navigatable device, which the first author helped design and develop, is the L'DISQ device, whose development and technique we will discuss in detail in the following sections.

The plasma-generating tissue ablation technique is well established and quantitatively adjustable to protect the delicate structures within the surgical field. We previously optimized a plasma generation instrument using a discharge tip made of stainless steel and samples of porcine nuclei [21]. We found that plasma discharge and tissue ablation occurred at the bubble's surface formed around the tip as the instrument was discharging. After approximately 300 s and vaporization of 1.35 g, the heated tip showed a focal accumulation of carbon.

The point of contact between the tip and tissue must be constantly changed to remove tissue and prevent carbonization, achieved by rotating, repositioning, and vibrating the catheter handle. By manipulating the catheter tip from the handle, we achieved optimal efficiency by moving the catheter handle at 2.5 mm/s with an output voltage of 280 V [22].

When accessing an extruded disc using an intradiscal approach, we found that the tip often could not be manipulated through the radial annular tear into the extrusion, especially when the tear and extrusion were not aligned. Furthermore, after bending the tip to redirect posteriorly, the forces on the catheter would tend to make it curl back rather than continue into the herniation.

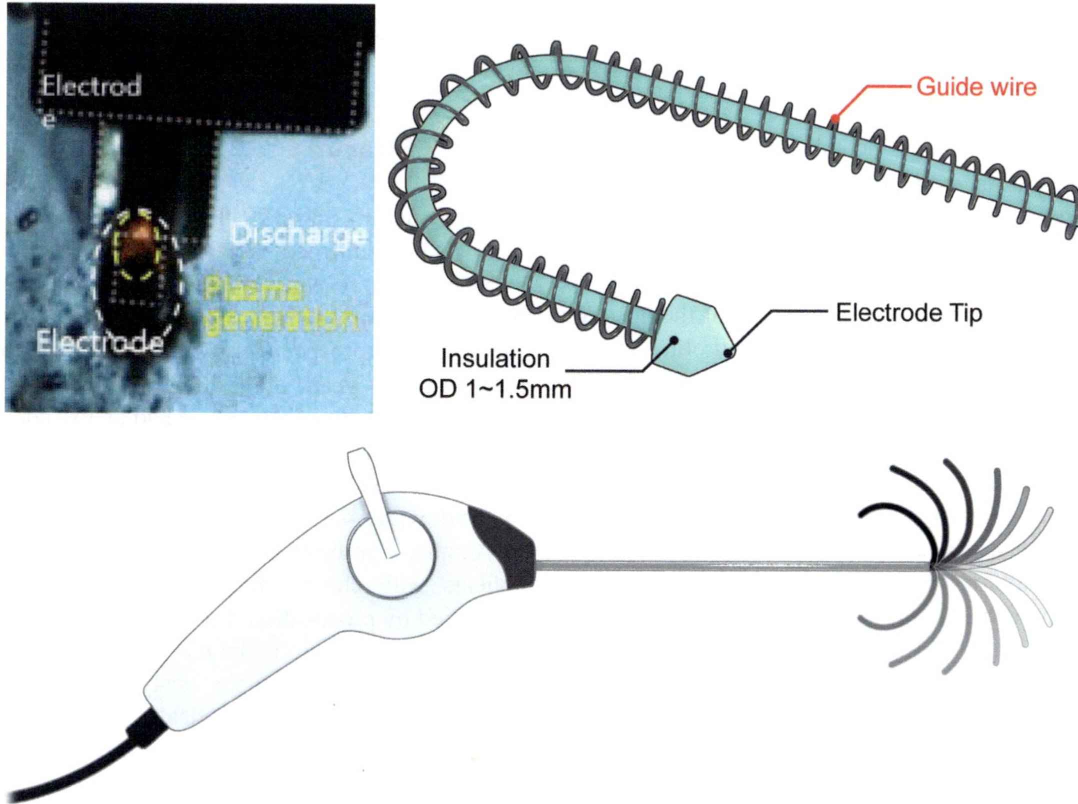

Fig. 8.1 Plasma-generating tissue ablation and proportional catheter navigation instrument

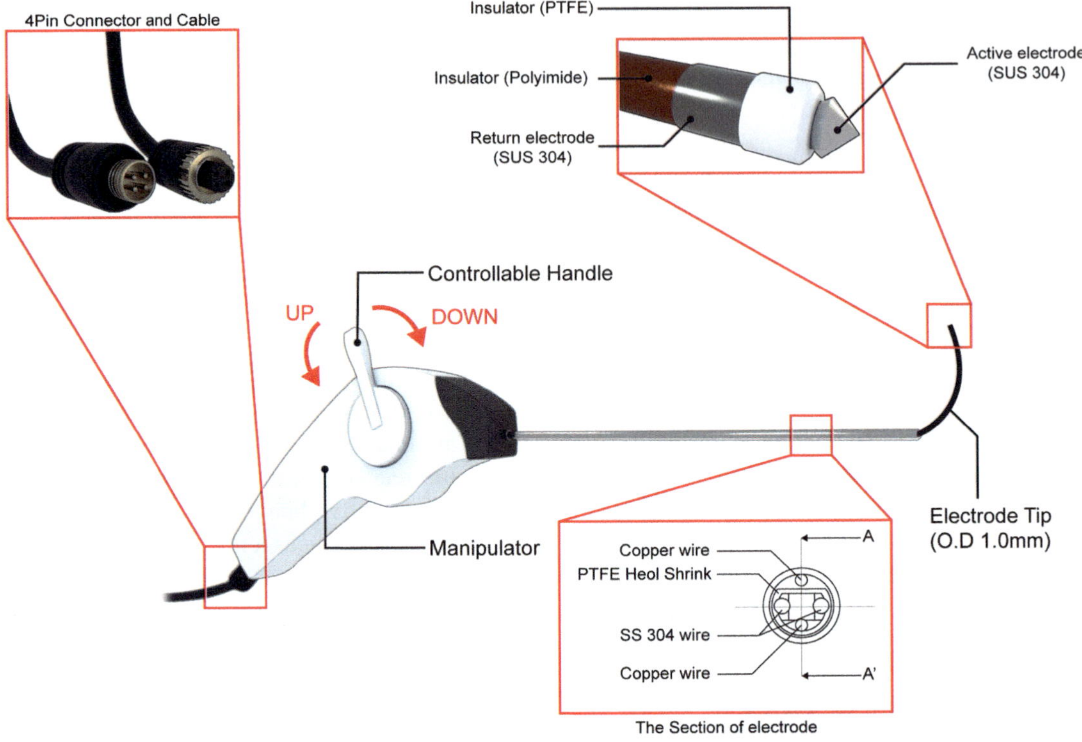

Fig. 8.2 L'DISQ catheter components

For both large contained and most noncontained disc herniations, we recommend a direct transforaminal approach to the base of the herniated disc [23]. At lumbar levels cephalad to L5–S1, approaching from the contralateral side facilitates horizontal penetration of the posterior annulus [23]. The steep angle and oblique angle typically required to approach the L5–S1 disc often prevent the passage of the catheter across the midline. Therefore, we recommend an ipsilateral approach with a slight bend placed on the guide needle to help direct the needle posteriorly and medially [23].

And for the cervical approach, the right-sided approach is used because the esophagus lies to the left in the lower neck. Pressure with the index and middle fingers to the space between the trachea and the medial border of the SCM (sternocleidomastoid). A 25 gauge, 2.5-in, spinal needle is used for the procedure and the needle should be sloped 30° to 40° angle in front of the index finger tip. Tip of the needle—in the center of the disc.

8.5 Efficacy

The first author's initial 2011 study of 27 patients with EMG-confirmed radiculopathy, 20 with extruded discs, revealed a significant decrease in pain intensity and function [3]. The same author subsequently prospectively followed up 170 patients for 2 years after disc decompression. Eighty-six percent of the cohort had an extruded disc. At a 2-year follow-up, 78.3% of the patients maintained over 50% improvement in leg pain intensity with a 4.7% recurrence rate [24].

Another preliminary study included 20 patients with chronic lumbar discogenic pain confirmed by provocation discography. In 20, we placed the catheter tip in the most prominent tear site identified by discographic analysis (Fig. 8.3). The clinical results were statistically significant at 48 weeks, but 20% of the patients had symptom recurrence 4–12 weeks after the procedure [25]. Unpublished data evaluation showed that the subjects' pain intensity was highly variable before the procedure, with significant differences between

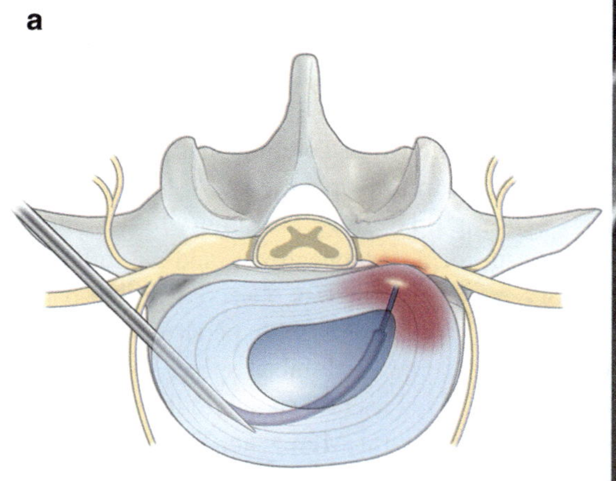

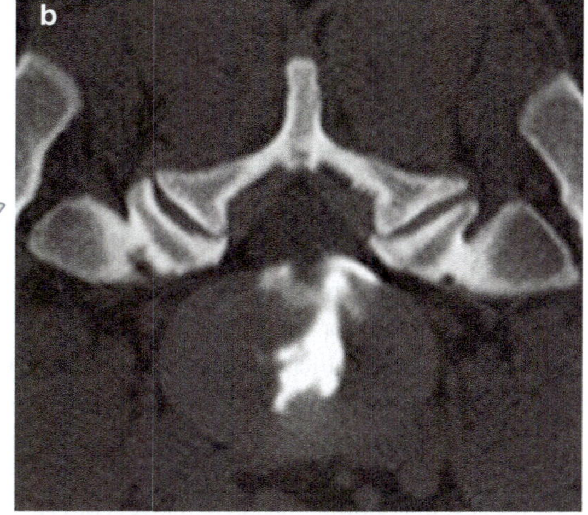

Fig. 8.3 A catheter applied to treat chronic lumbar discogenic pain and a discogram at the same level. The figures present a schematic diagram (**b**) in which a catheter that has entered from the contralateral side is bent and progressed within the annular fissure (**a**) identified in the CT discogram

groups with and without pain improvement. In some cases, a numeric rating scale of 10/10 VAS fell to zero after 12 weeks of treatment while in others, an intensity of three before the procedure worsened to six 12 weeks postoperatively. We were unable to predict prognosis based on preprocedural variables. We attribute our inconsistent results to persistent inflammation caused by retained dead and dying nuclear materials incompletely removed during the procedure.

For cervical decompression with percutaneous navigable wand, pilot study was conducted with 20 consecutive patients, 12 males and 8 females with a mean age of 45.4 years ranging from 28 to 65 years. The mean duration of symptoms was 5.6 months with a range of 1–20 months. The level of the targeted disc was as follows; C3/4 in 1 patient, C4/5 in 2 patients, C5/6 in 6 patients, and C6/7 in 11 patients. The disc protrusion was demonstrated in 10 patients, and the disc extrusion was demonstrated in other 10 patients according to the MRI readings.

Following the procedure, serial follow-up clinical data were obtained for all 20 patients for 48 weeks. Compared to the preoperative baseline, the NRS, NDI, and SF-36 BP scores showed statistical improvement at the postoperative 48 weeks follow-up. The average reported pain level as measured by NRS was 7 before the procedure and 1 after 48 weeks postprocedure. There was significant NRS improvement for the first 4 weeks ($p = 0.01$) after the procedure. No further meaningful improvement was reported from 4 weeks to 48 weeks, but the initial improvement was sustained. NDI decreased significantly for 1 week postoperatively ($p = 0.01$), and continued improving until 48 weeks, from 44 to 9 points. The SF-36 BP scale increased significantly for 1 week postoperatively compared to the baseline of 33.20 ($p = 0.02$), and improved steadily to 51 at 48 weeks. Successful outcomes were reported in 16 patients (80.0%), with a reduction of NRS by more than 50%. Four subjects did not show any successful outcomes. One subject showed NRS decrement until post-24 weeks, but the symptom recurred between 24 and 48 weeks. The other three patients recorded incorrect tip placement. On post-procedural CT images, some radiolucent spots were often identified in epidural and targeted intervertebral space, which were presumed to be vaporized air bubbles. The bony structures and alignments were scanned and compared with pre-procedural MRI or simple X-ray images, but no specific changes were observed in any of the patients.

The final placement of the wand tip was confirmed by fluoroscopic AP and lateral views in all participants. The wand was passed beyond the disc margin and into the disc herniation. The location of the wand tip resulted in 16 correct and 4 incorrect placements. The wand tips of all incorrect cases were placed on more inner side beneath the herniated base. Therefore, the tip could not approach the target area from the center of the disc. Unsuccessful outcomes were reported in 4 cases, 3 incorrect and 1 correct tip case, at post-48 weeks which showed a significant correlation between correct tip placements and successful outcomes after 48 weeks.

The limitation of this study was that it was a pilot study with a short-term follow-up and few subjects. A randomized and controlled-study is required in the future. Comparisons of the clinical efficacy, depending on cervical levels or types of herniation, would be needed to ascertain the application of the percutaneous disc decompression with the navigable wand on various patients with cervical HNP. Despite these limitations, the promising results and safety of the procedure in this study encourages us to utilize this technique in well-selected cases.

8.6 Complications

A few patients (5.7%, $n = 11/192$) reported discomfort and sensory abnormalities consistent with a radicular pattern lasting 1 to 3 months. However, 1.6% of the patients ($n = 3/192$) developed a foot drop. In one case, marked axonal injury of an L5 root was associated with muscle weakness lasting over 1 year [24]. In this case, hot saline leaked from the intervertebral disc during procedure, resulting in thermal damage to the nerve. After rehabilitation, all three patients recovered to a fair grade of dorsiflexion of the foot. Therefore, continuous infusion of saline to promote plasma generation is strongly discouraged due to the potential for thermal nerve damage. The distance between the nerve tissue and the tip of the L'DISQ wand may be reduced during tissue removal even if the tip position is correct, especially where extruded materials are closely attached to the root or nerve in the absence of even a thin outer annulus. If the wand's tip is near the nerve tissue for a prolonged period, electrical stimulation resulting in a thermal axonal injury is possible.

For the cervical pilot study, no intra-procedure or post-procedure complications were reported such as swallowing discomfort, hoarseness, esophageal perforation, vascular or nerve injuries, infection and cerebrospinal fluid leakage, during the follow-up period.

During tip heating, heat injury to the endplate caused local osteonecrosis, and an inflammatory bone reaction was observed in one patient. In other 10 patients with persistent axial pain (cervical spine, 3; lumbar spine, 7), a radiologist diagnosed aseptic spondylodiscitis based on a post-procedural MRI scan. Endplate injury is preventable [26].

8.7 Procedural Protocol

Step 1 Preoperative

1. Review history and imaging.
2. Allergic skin test for antibiotics (optional).
3. Intravenous antibiotics 30 min before the procedure.

Step 2 Preparation

- *Lumbar*
  1. Abdominal pillow-supported prone position.
  2. Real-time vital sign monitoring by qualified personnel.
  3. Mark the anatomical landmarks on the skin, including the vertebral endplates, pedicle, spinous process, iliac crest.
  4. Surgical drapes.
  5. Follow global guidelines for preventing surgical site infection (World Health Organization. Global guidelines for preventing surgical site infection. World Health Organization, 2016.)
- *Cervical*
  1. Supine position with the neck extended gently by placing a cushion beneath the shoulder and gently distract both shoulders downward to the operation table
  2. Place the soft strap over the forehead for stabilization.
  3. Real-time monitoring system for vital signs

4. Mark the anatomical landmarks on the skin including the vertebral endplates, pedicle, spinous process, iliac crest
5. Surgical drapes
6. Follow global guidelines for preventing surgical site infection (World Health Organization. Global guidelines for preventing surgical site infection. World Health Organization, 2016.)

Step 3 Demark the Target Disc Outer Annulus

1. This is a step that is usually not performed, though not wholly unnecessary. Perform discogram using a 25-gauge needle, injecting 1 to 2 mL of contrast to outline the disc herniation. However, ionized contrast media commonly used in spinal procedures prevent plasma generation during the procedure, so this step is often skipped.
2. Document that disc outlined on the lateral C-arm view (Fig. 8.4).

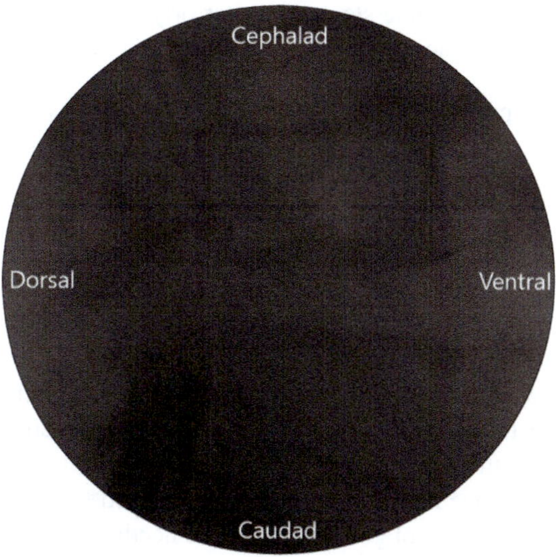

Fig. 8.4 Demark the target disc outer annulus

Step 4 Skin Entry Site

- *Lumbar*
  1. Using fluoroscopy, select a point 12–15 cm laterally from the spinous process midline of the target IVD under fluoroscopic guidance.
  2. Inject local anesthetization of the skin, fascia, and muscle layers.
  3. The puncture point is slightly anterior to the SAP visualized in an ipsilateral oblique C-arm projection of approximately 15°. The SAP should be approximately 3/5 across the anterior-posterior vertebral body distance with the endplates aligned (Figs. 8.5 and 8.6).
- *Cervical*
  1. Commonly the approach is made on the right side of the patient because the esophagus lies to the left in the lower neck (Fig. 8.7).

     (However, in the right posterolateral or foraminal cervical HNP, the left approach may be considered with extra caution not to injure the esophagus.)
  2. Select a point by touching the target disc with the tip of two fingers.
  3. Inject local anesthetization of the skin, fascia, and muscle layers.
  4. Press firmly with the index and middle fingers to the space between the trachea and the medial border of the SCM (sternocleido-

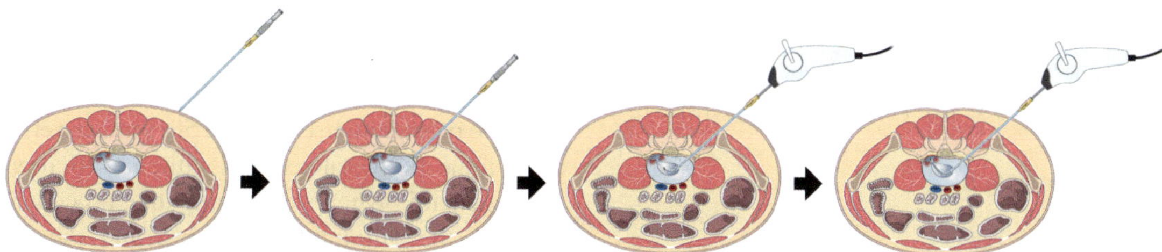

Fig. 8.5 The skin entering point is about 8 to 10 cm laterally from the spinous process midline of the target IVD under fluoroscopic guidance. The puncture point is slightly anterior to the SAP visualized in an ipsilateral oblique C-arm projection of approximately 30°

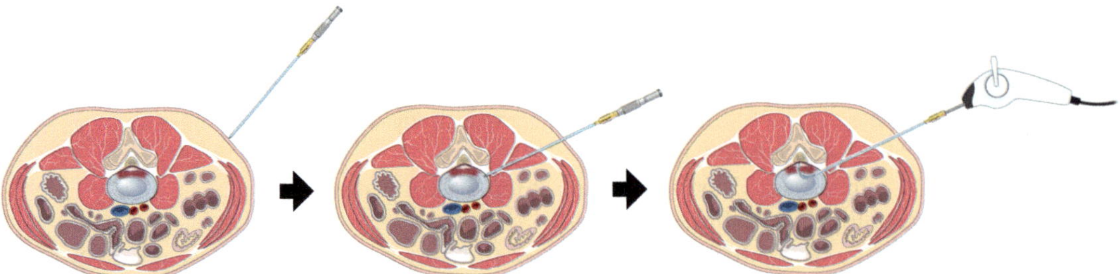

Fig. 8.6 The skin entry point is around the lateral margin of the quadratus lumborum, a muscle that is the most lateral side of the back muscle. This entering point is about 12 to 15 cm laterally from the spinous process midline of the target IVD under fluoroscopic guidance. The puncture point is slightly anterior to the SAP visualized in an ipsilateral oblique C-arm projection of approximately 60~75°

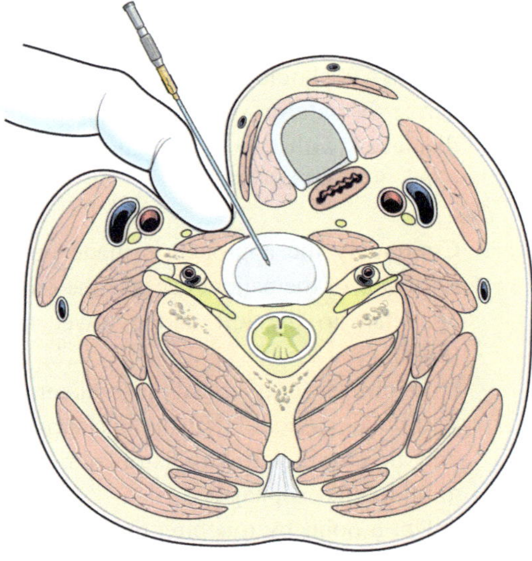

Fig. 8.7 Press firmly with the index and middle fingers to the space between the trachea and the medial border of the SCM (sternocleidomastoid), pushing trachea and esophagus toward the central direction simultaneously

mastoid), pushing trachea and esophagus toward the central direction simultaneously.

5. A 25 gauge, 2.5-in, spinal needle is punctured between two fingers' tip with 30° to 40° angle in the view of a fluoroscopy rotated 15° from a vertical projection.

Step 5 Approach

– *Lumbar*

1. In the AP view, the introducer needle is directed down the beam toward a contact point at the disc margin at a line drawn between the medial borders of adjacent pedicles.
2. A "corkscrew" rotation of the slightly curved distal tip is used, directing the introducer needle toward the lateral edge of the SAP. Manually forming a gentle curve on the needle length will also later facilitate steerage posteriorly into the disc or across the midline outside the disc.

- The access procedure for plasma decompression of the lumbar 4–5 level is not difficult to perform.

The most difficult level of this procedure is the intervertebral space between the 5th lumbar vertebra and the 1st sacrum. It is very convenient to perform the procedure when the tip of the trocar is bent about 15° by about 8–10 mm from the distal end, as if one were driving in the direction that they want.

A needle with a curved tip is pushed forward, and instead of going straight, the needle moves in the bent direction.

As if driving, if you rotate the needle in the direction where the tip of the needle is bent and then driven forward, you can easily position it where you want it to go. Since it is easy to adjust the direction of the needle, it is possible to perform the procedure between the 5th lumbar vertebra and the 1st sacral vertebra without difficulty.

In general, when performing the procedure between the 5th lumbar vertebra and the 1st sacrum, a needle is inserted between the iliac crest and the vertebrae to avoid the pelvic bone. In this case, the angle between the anteroposterior line of the vertebral body and the needle is so narrow that it is very difficult to position the tip of the trocar on the back of the disc or on the torn posterior annulus.

It is good to start the procedure for lumbar 5—sacral 1 at the same needle puncture location as for 4–5 lumbar vertebrae. In the procedure of the bending needle, it is advantageous that the starting point is as far from the spine as possible.

It is better to start at the lateral end of the muscle that is palpable by palpation of the paravertebral muscle. This site is the postoerolateral area of the trunk and is located more than 12 cm lateral from the spinous process of the vertebral body.

Step 6 Contact and Advance

1. Touch the lateral SAP edge and then direct the needle tip over the process with the curve pointing away from the midline. Once over the SAP, the operator typically rotates the needle to point toward the midline.
2. Do not puncture the normal posterior annulus if it is probable that one can directly puncture a central HNP or the target is a contralateral extrusion.
3. Advancement slowly using the lateral image with intermediate AP and lateral views. Both the distal bend and optional long gentle curve facilitate precise directional control by needle rotation.
4. The annulus is typically felt and confirmed by AP and lateral C-arm views. Typically one will feel a loss of resistance when the outer annulus is punctured.
5. Check the AP view before slowly advancing into the nucleus but typically advance using the lateral view. The needle tip should not be beyond the medial border of the pedicle (Fig. 8.8).

- *Cervical*
    1. The needle is inserted toward the center of the disc.
    2. After the needle penetrates the annulus, advance less than 5 mm further to avoid the needle being pulled out due to disc pressure.
    3. 3, Place the needle in the posterior 1/3 of the disc, checking with lateral view of C-ARM.
    4. Fix the trocar needle is with sterile surgical tape.

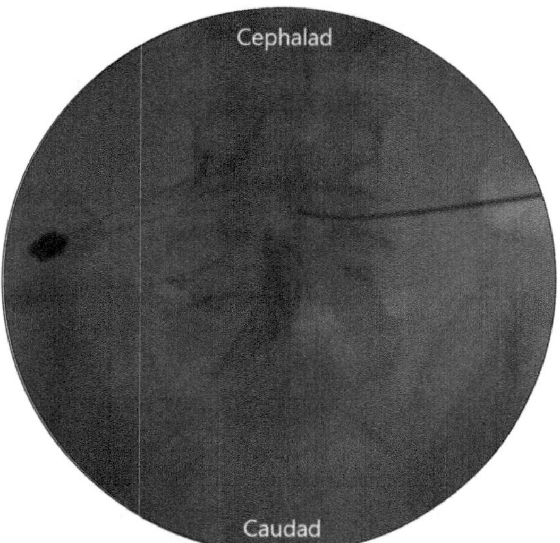

Fig. 8.8 Placement

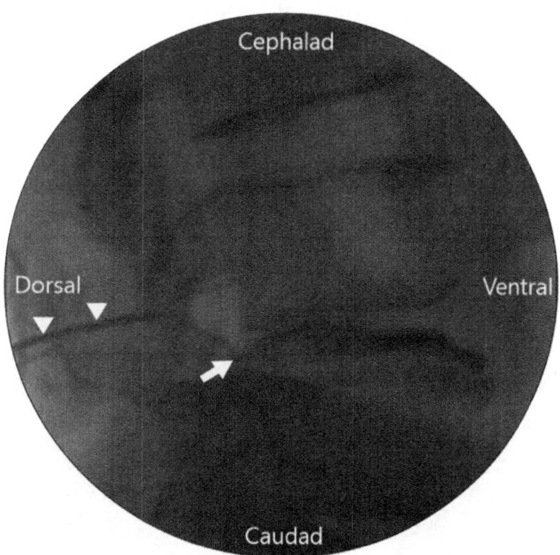

Fig. 8.9 The location of the tip just before ablation. Arrow heads indicate the L'disq wand, and the arrow indicates the location of herniated disc

Step 7 Wand Placement

1. After confirming nuclear placement or placement in a central or extruded disc, remove the stylet and replace with the wand.
2. Before ablation, confirm a negative motor nerve stimulation with 2–3 volts at 2 hertz (Fig. 8.9). Doublecheck the needle position when the tip lies in a herniated disc.

Similarly to the existing intradiscal procedure, once the distal end of the plasma wand is placed into the nucleus pulposus, the ruptured annulus tissue is degenerated, an effect caused by the plasma wand inevitably passing through the disc. While this direct approach is a difficult method, if the distal end of the plasma wand is directly approached from the epidural space into the prolapsed disc tissue, the prolapsed disc can be effectively removed without degenerative changes in the normal disc tissue. Before the procedure is performed, on the MRI image taken, the exact prolapse of the nucleus pulposus of the disc is checked and the procedure is executed.

The following procedure must be executed with extreme caution so as to avoid damaging the nerve. The location of the trocar should be located at the center of the posterior annulus on the posterior vertebral margin line in the lateral view of the C-arm. Afterwards, it should be placed at the center of the protruded disc confirmed by MRI in the A-P view. After the trocar reaches the desired position, remove the metal guide needle of the trocar. Slowly insert the plasma wand into the remaining polymer sheath (Fig. 8.10).

If the distal end of the wand is located inside the prolapsed disc, it does not advance further because it touches the wall of the annulus fibrosus; the surgeon cannot advance the wand into the surgical site any farther without applying excessive force. If the distal end of the wand continues to progress past the lesion identified in the C-arm images, this may be indication that it has escaped into the epidural space or is incorrectly positioned.

In this case, it is also possible to obtain more precise information by injecting contrast media into the epidural space. In addition, when electrical stimulation is applied in the nerve stimulation mode, the nerve is stimulated, muscle contraction occurs in the lower extremities, and the patient feels the electrical stimulation.

- *Cervical*
  1. A navigable wand is inserted after removing the guide needle.
  2. Adjust the position of the wand tip to the torn annulus using AP-lateral view of C-ARM.

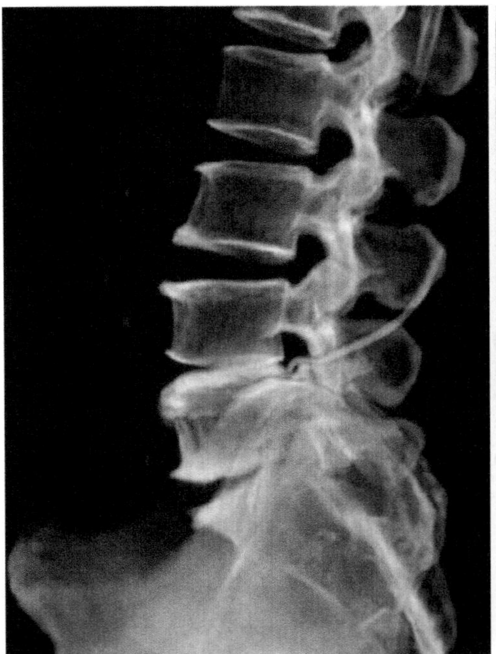
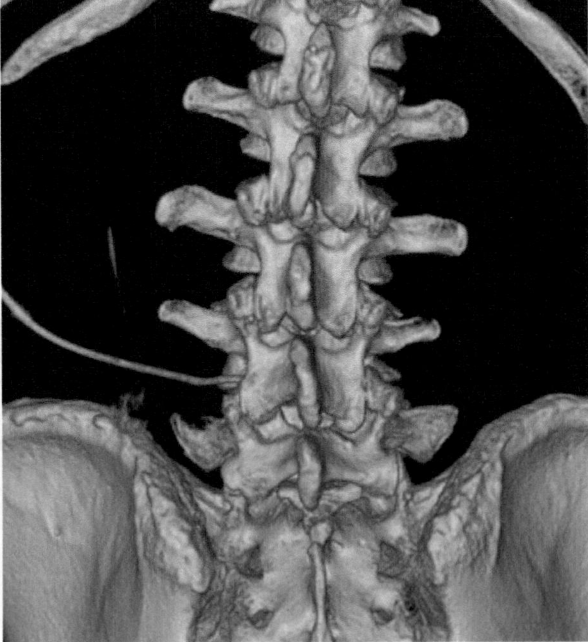

Fig. 8.10 These images show the pathway of L'DISQ wand by 3D reconstruction of CT images taken during the L'disq procedure. It can be seen that the path of the wand went directly into the prolapsed nucleus pulposus without passing through the normal annulus fibrosus. While this direct approach is a difficult method, he prolapsed disc can be effectively removed without degenerative changes in the normal disc tissue

3. Change the patient's neck to a flexion position to secure a space to enter the torn annulus and insert the wand with gentle pressure.
4. the wand does not enter the torn annulus with gentle pressure, check the tip position with AP-lateral view and activate the plasma ablation several times around the torn annulus. (Plasma can remove the nucleus pulposus containing water components, but not the annulus. Therefore, removing the nucleus pulposus that blocks the tear with plasma ablation allows the entry through the torn annulus.)

- The entry of the tip should be done only with gentle pressure and the plasma ablation must be turned off before entering to prevent nerve damage.

Step 8 Ablation

1. Make sure the patient is awake and can report pain. Able for 5 s, repeatedly checking a negative nerve stimulation (Fig. 8.11).
2. Rotate or reposition to prevent stagnation of the contact surface between the tissue and the tip during ablation.
3. The total ablation time is typically between 150 and 300 s for lumbar discs and between 120 and 200 s for cervical discs.
4. Make sure nerve stimulation is negative before each 5-s ablation.
5. To prevent local heat accumulation, slowly inject intermittent 0.5 to 1 ml boluses of room temperature or cold normal saline using a 25G spinal needle located in the safety zone of the epidural space (Fig. 8.12).
6. It is recommended to stop after performing additional ablation of 20–30 s after the patient's neurological symptoms have improved.

- Plasma decompression is a procedure that improves the patient's symptoms by removing a part of the herniated disc and then helps additional recovery through rehabilitation treatment of the core muscle. Therefore, it is better not to try to remove all the herniated disc with plasma ablation.
- If the nerve is stimulated, it means that the distal end of the wand is in very approximate contact with the nerve. At this time, if nerve stimulation does not occur again, ablation is performed again because there is a safe loca-

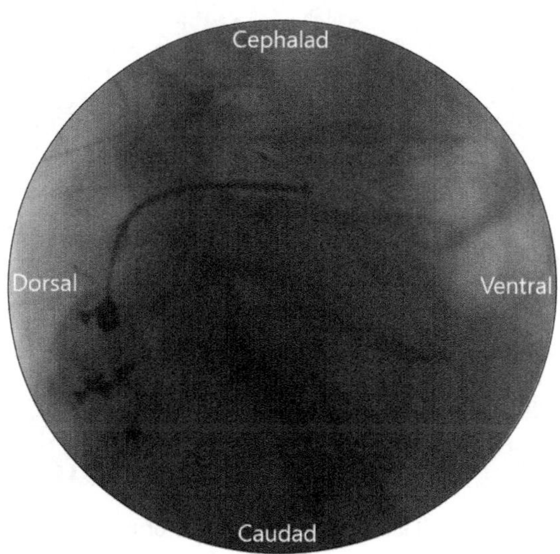

Fig. 8.11 Ablation

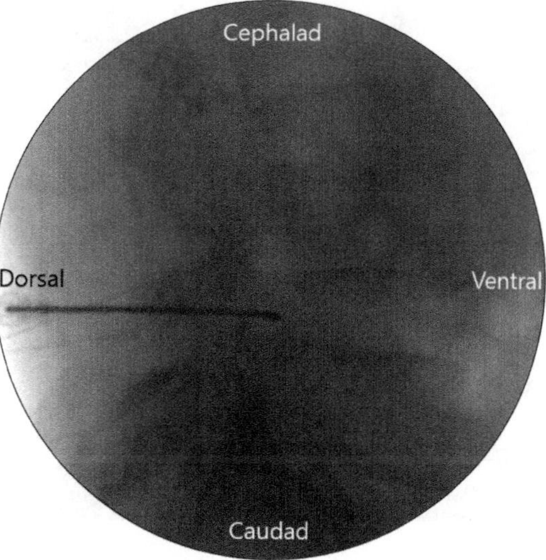

Fig. 8.12 Lateral view of the wand and spinal needle placement during ablation

tion. If the nerve is stimulated during ablation, the procedure must be aborted immediately and repositioned. When the prolapsed disc tissue is successfully removed, the tip of the wand and the nerve are positioned very close to each other with a thin annulus fibrosus in between, and weak nerve stimulation symptoms appear. The patient begins to feel miniscule electrical stimulation, and during the procedure, the patient's minute muscle contractions can be observed in the back or buttock muscle. In this case, if the ablation is stopped immediately and the position is adjusted, the procedure can be completed relatively safely. Therefore, it is necessary to alert the patient to notify the medical staff immediately if there is even a mild electrical stimulation before the procedure. If there is weak nerve stimulation, stop the ablation, adjust the position of the wand, and then repeat the ablation.

Step 9 Coagulation

1. After ablation, maneuver the tip into the middle of the annular fissure and after changing to coagulation mode, coagulate for 10–15 s, again with intermittent stimulation.

Step 10 Tip Removal

1. Remove instruments in the following order: the catheter, introducer sheath, and 25G spinal needle (Fig. 8.8).
2. Partial compressive dressing of the skin entry site.
3. Check for bleeding.

Step 11 Postoperative Care

1. Can obtain a baseline post-procedure Image scan (CT or MRI) (Fig. 8.13), if physician wants to check the amount of decompression or to evaluate possible structural complications after intervention, etc.

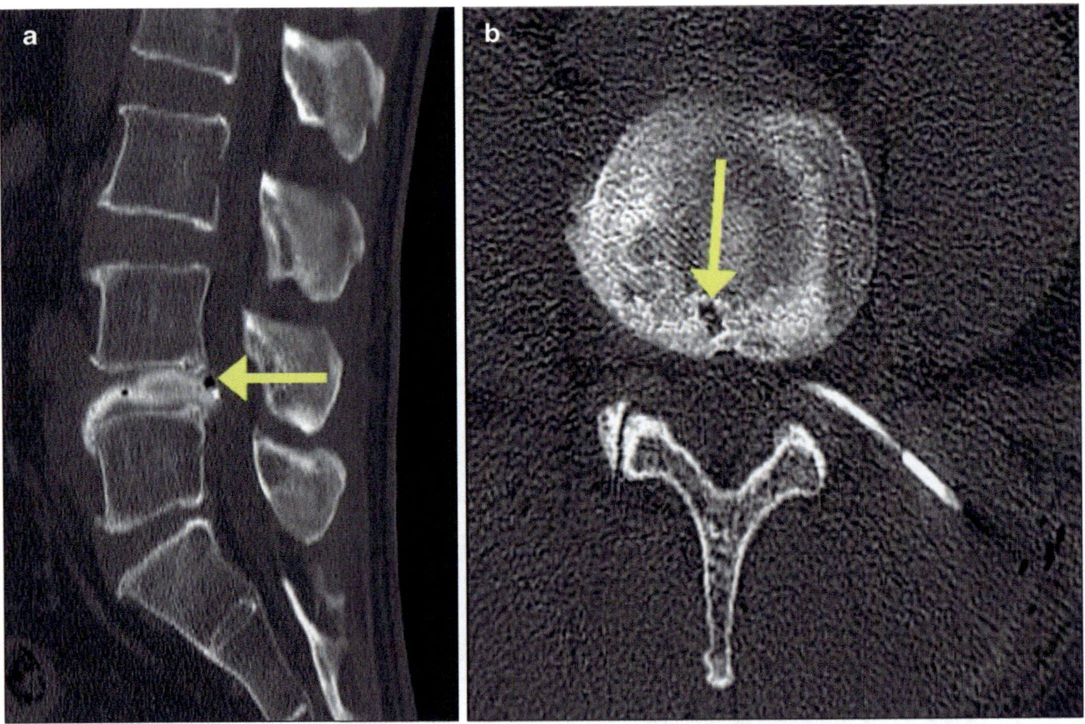

Fig. 8.13 Postoperative computed tomographic scan. The yellow arrow indicates the ablation site of the disc tissue after the procedure

2. Absolute bed rest on supine position for 4 h post-procedure.
3. Use routine surgical wound care.
4. Assess the pain intensity on the next day.

8.8 Conclusions

Percutaneous options to decompress a herniated disc are rapidly evolving. While current catheter-directed ablative technologies can effectively treat radicular pain caused by a herniated disc, consistent treatment of axial pain remains suboptimal.

References

1. Hijikata S. Percutaneous nucleotomy. A new concept technique and 12 years experience. Clin Orthop Relat Res. 1989;238:9–23.
2. Singh V, Manchikanti L, Benyamin RM, Helm S, Hirsch JA. Percutaneous lumbar laser disc decompression: a systematic review of current evidence. Pain Physician. 2009;12:573–88.
3. Lee SH, Derby R, Sul D, Hong J, Kim GH, Kang S, et al. Efficacy of a new navigable percutaneous disc decompression device (L'DISQ) in patients with herniated nucleus pulposus related to radicular pain. Pain Med. 2011;12:370–6.
4. Kambin P. Percutaneous lumbar discectomy—indication, technique and results. In: Mayer HM, Brock M, editors. Percutaneous lumbar discectomy. New York City: Springer; 1989. p. 87–93.
5. Helms CA, Onik G, Davis GW. Automated percutaneous lumbar discectomy. Skelet Radiol. 1989;18:579–83.
6. Manchikanti L, Singh V, Falco FJE, Calodney AK, Onyewu O, Helm S 2nd, et al. An updated review of automated percutaneous mechanical lumbar discectomy for the contained herniated lumbar disc. Pain Physician. 2013;16(2 Suppl):SE151–84.
7. Hirsch JA, Singh V, Falco FJE, Benyamin RM, Manchikanti L. Automated percutaneous lumbar discectomy for the contained herniated lumbar disc: a systematic assessment of evidence. Pain Physician. 2009;12:601–20.
8. Sim SE, Ko ES, Kim DK, Kim HK, Kim YC, Shin HY. The results of cervical nucleoplasty in patients with cervical disc disorder: a retrospective clinical study of 22 patients. Korean J Pain. 2011;24(1):36–43.
9. Eichen PM, Achilles N, Konig V, Mosges R, Hellmich M, Himpe B, et al. Nucleoplasty, a minimally invasive procedure for disc decompression: a systematic review and meta-analysis of published clinical studies. Pain Physician. 2014;17:E149–73.
10. Bokov A, Isrelov A, Skorodumov A, Aleynik A, Simonov A, Mlyavykh S. An analysis of reasons for failed back surgery syndrome and partial results after different types of surgical lumbar nerve root decompression. Pain Physician. 2011;14:545–57.
11. Sharps LS, Isaac Z. Percutaneous disc decompression using nucleoplasty. Pain Physician. 2002;5:121–6.
12. Schenk B, Brouwer PA, Peul WC, van Buchem MA. Percutaneous laser disk decompression: a review of the literature. AJNR Am J Neuroradiol. 2006;27:232–5.
13. Choi JY, Tanenbaum BS, Milner TE, Dao XV, Nelson JS, Sobol EN, Wong BJ. Theramal, mechanical, optical, and morphologic changes in bovine nucleus pulposus induced by Nd:YAG (λ= 1.32 μm) laser irradiation. Lasers Surg Med. 2001;28(3):248–54.
14. Nygaard OP, Mellgren SI, Osterud B. The inflammatory properties of contained and noncontained lumbar disc herniation. Spine (Phila Pa 1976). 1997;22:2484–8.
15. Haro H, Shinomiya K, Komori H, Okawa A, Saito I, Miyasaka N, et al. Upregulated expression of chemokines in herniated nucleus pulposus resorption. Spine (Phila Pa 1976). 1996;21:1647–52.
16. Fardon DF, Milette PC. Nomenclature and classification of lumbar disc pathology. Recommendations of the combined task forces of the North American Spine Society, American Society of Spine Radiology, and American Society of Neuroradiology. Spine (Phila Pa 1976). 2001;26:E93–113.
17. Weiner BK, Patel R. The accuracy of MRI in the detection of lumbar disc containment. J Orthop Surg Res. 2008;3:46.
18. Takahashi K, Miyazaki T, Takino T, Matsui T, Tomita K. Epidural pressure measurements. Relationship between epidural pressure and posture in patients with lumbar spinal stenosis. Spine (Phila Pa 1976). 1995;20:650–3.
19. Takahashi K, Kagechika K, Takino T, Matsui T, Miyazaki T, Shima I. Changes in epidural pressure during walking in patients with lumbar spinal stenosis. Spine (Phila Pa 1976). 1995;20:2746–9.
20. Sato K, Kikuchi S, Yonezawa T. In vivo intradiscal pressure measurement in healthy individuals and in patients with ongoing back problems. Spine (Phila Pa 1976). 1999;24:2468–74.
21. Lee SH, Kim NH, Kim GH, Bae B, Shin JS, Park SS, et al. Characteristics of molybdenum as a plasma-generating electrode. Sci Adv Mater. 2016;8:1844–7.
22. Yoon SY, Kim GH, Kim Y, Kim NH, Lee S, Kawai C, et al. Optimal parameters for intervertebral disk resection using aqua-plasma beams. J Neurol Surg A Cent Eur Neurosurg. 2019;80:34–8.
23. Lee SC, Lee SH. The navigable percutaneous disc decompression device (L'DISQ & L'DISQ-C) in patients with herniated nucleus pulposus related to radicular pain. In: Pain and treatment IntechOpen. 2014.

24. Kim NH, Hong Y, Lee SH. Two-year clinical outcomes of radiofrequency focal ablation using a navigable plasma disc decompression device in patients with lumbar disc herniation: efficacy and complications. J Pain Res. 2018;11:2229–37.
25. Lee SH, Derby R, Sul D, Hong YK, Ha KW, Suh D, et al. Effectiveness of a new navigable percutaneous disc decompression device (L'DISQ) in patients with lumbar discogenic pain. Pain Med. 2015;16:266–73.
26. Yudoyono F, Kim DY, Chin DK, Shin DA. Aseptic spondylodiscitis resulting from intradiscal radiofrequency ablation (IDRA) in patients with herniated disc disease: a report of ten cases. J Minim Invasive Spine Surg Tech. 2018;3:13–7.

9 Transforaminal Discoplasty with Endoscopy

Jongsun Lee

9.1 Introduction

Diagnosing discogenic LBP is often difficult, and localizing the exact pain generator is not possible in many cases. The treatment of annulogenic, discogenic LBP is still challenging because of the limited healing capacity of the AF and proximity of the torn AF to neural structures. Various intra- and extradiscal minimally invasive interventions have been introduced to avoid surgery-related problems; however, neither approach alone seems sufficient for success because each has limitations and risks.

New techniques that combine transforaminal epiduroscopy with advanced laser technologies have recently become a focus of attention. Direct visualization of spinal canal pathoanatomy and reproduction of the patient's usual pain by directly stimulating the suspected pain generator under endoscopic guidance improve diagnostic accuracy substantially. The precise application of a laser under direct vision greatly enhances the safety and efficacy of discoplasty.

Percutaneous endoscopic lumbar annuloplasty and nucleoplasty (PELAN) is an intra-annular procedure that directly targets the granulation tissue in the torn AF. Transforaminal epiduroscopic laser annuloplasty (TELA) is essentially an extradiscal procedure intended to denervate the sensitized nociceptive nerves in the posterior AF, and simultaneous intradiscal ablation can be performed if needed. Transforaminal epiduroscopic laser discoplasty might be a reasonable second-line treatment option for annulogenic, discogenic LBP.

9.2 Background

Usually, most people who experience LBP recover in a week or two. However, recurrence is common, and for some people, LBP can become chronic and disabling. Reportedly, an IVD is the cause of symptoms in 26–42% of patients with chronic LBP [1, 2]. The peripheral AF and endplates are richly innervated, and they can be important pain generators [3]. Discogenic LBP pain can be classified into two types according to the pain generator: annular disruption-induced (i.e., annulogenic) pain and endplate disruption-induced pain [4] (Fig. 9.1). These two types of discogenic LBP cannot be differentiated clinically. Internal disc disruption (IDD), first described by Crock [4], can also be categorized into two types according to the pain generator:

Supplementary Information The online version contains supplementary material available at [https://doi.org/10.1007/978-981-16-9547-6_9].

J. Lee (✉)
Department of Neurosurgery, Nasaret International Hospital, Incheon, Republic of Korea

S.-H. Lee (ed.), *Minimally Invasive Spine Interventions*, https://doi.org/10.1007/978-981-16-9547-6_9

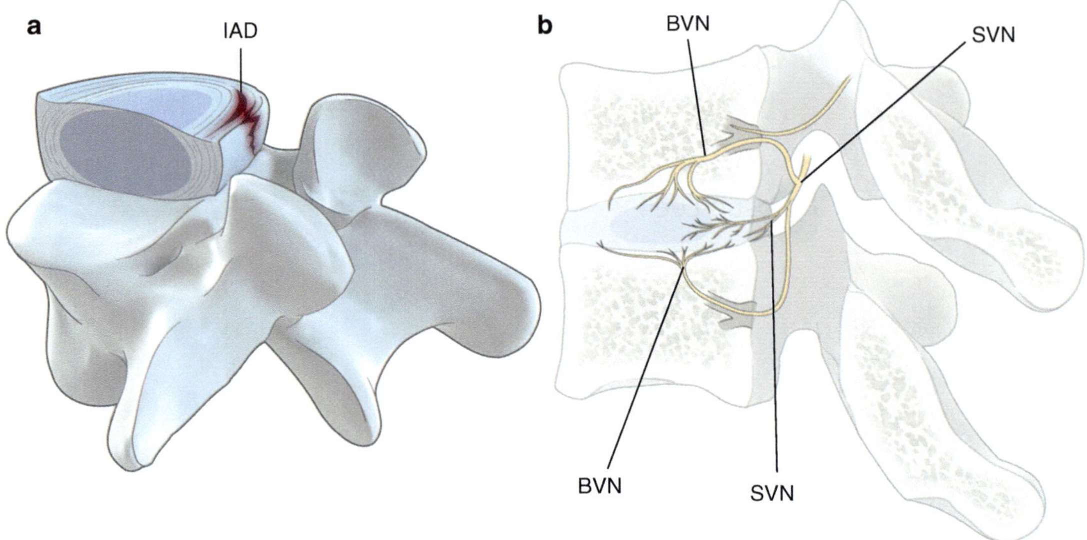

Fig. 9.1 Classification of discogenic low back pain according to the pain generator: annular disruption-induced (i.e., annulogenic) pain and endplate disruption-induced pain. Internal annular disruption can causes annulogenic, discogenic low back pain (**a**). The posterior annulus fibrosus is innervated by sinuvertebral nerve. The endplates are innervated by basivertebral nerves. IAD, internal annular disruption; BVN, basivertebral nerve; SVN, sinuvertebral nerve

internal annular disruption (IAD) and internal endplate disruption (IED).

The pathological process of IAD usually begins with AF tearing. The formation and propagation of annular tears, subsequent ingrowth of nociceptive nerves and vascular granulation tissues in the AF, sensitization of the nociceptors, and epidural inflammation secondary to leakage of nuclear materials are considered the key mechanisms of annulogenic, discogenic LBP [2].

Despite the availability of modern diagnostic tools, the precise anatomical location of persistent LBP is often difficult to identify. The most commonly used method for diagnosing discogenic LBP is MRI. A high-intensity zone (HIZ) on T2-weighted MRI is a typical finding in an annular tear [5]. An HIZ associated with an annular tear contains both trapped intra-annular nuclear material and inflamed granulation tissue. However, MRI cannot definitively demonstrate whether a disc is painful. Some annular tears are asymptomatic healed lesions, and some are not visible.

Provocative discography is a practical test for the identification of discogenic LBP [6]. However, due to the poor specificity of discography, the test's clinical utility and diagnostic accuracy are questionable, and the procedure may damage the disc and promote disc degeneration. Further, even using provocative discography, the exact site of the pain generator is not easily identified. Therefore, a more specific and reliable test is required to localize the pain generator accurately, and direct disc stimulation is an effective option. Similar to palpation during a physical examination, the operator can directly stimulate the annular surface with a probe during open surgery or transforaminal epiduroscopy. A study of the pain response to tissue stimulation during lumbar spine surgery under local anesthesia demonstrated that the posterior AF was the most common site of back pain reproduction [7]. Approximately two-thirds of the patients experienced pain with direct mechanical stimulation of the outer AF with blunt surgical instruments or an electrical current. Moderate LBP and severe concordant pain were each perceived by one-third of the patients. During transforaminal epiduroscopy, probing the torn AF can provoke concordant pain in the patient. Pain provocation by annular stimulation before, and diminished tenderness after, laser denervation might be definitive evidence of annulogenic, discogenic LBP.

Discogenic LBP is typically managed using a stepladder approach to treatment, ranging from conservative therapy to minimally invasive spinal intervention to invasive surgical treatment such as discectomy, artificial disc replacement, or spinal fusion. Surgery is associated with risks, complications, and prolonged recovery.

To avoid surgery-related problems, various minimally invasive interventional procedures that use either the caudal or transforaminal route have been developed as second-line treatments, and their number continues to increase [8]. These techniques include epidural adhesiolysis (neuroplasty), percutaneous disc decompression procedures (automated percutaneous lumbar discectomy [APLD], percutaneous laser disc decompression [PLDD], Dekompressor [Stryker Corp., Kalamazoo, MI, US], disc nucleoplasty, and others), and percutaneous thermal intradiscal procedures (intradiscal electrothermal therapy [IDET], DiscTRODE [Radionics, Burlington, MA, US], biacuplasty, Disc-Fx [Elliquence, Baldwin, NY, US], L'DISQ, and others). There is considerable controversy over the efficacy of these therapies. All percutaneous intradiscal procedures are image-guided blind techniques that the outermost layer of the posterior AF can not be easily denervated, often resulting in insufficient treatment of pain. Further, they carry the risk of thermal neural injury. Percutaneous or endoscopic epidural neuroplasty through the trans-sacral route is an easy and less invasive way to obtain ventral epidural extradiscal access [9–11]. Since the annular surface is only approached tangentially and an end-firing laser cannot penetrate the AF easily, this method seems unsuitable for intradiscal access.

The main goals of minimally invasive interventional treatments for annulogenic, discogenic LBP are pain relief and healing of the damaged disc (Fig. 9.2). Sensitized ingrown nociceptive nerves should be destroyed or denervated, from both inside and outside the AF, to eliminate pain. Herniated or interposed nuclear materials and ingrown granulation tissue in the AF should be removed while preserving and repairing the disc structure as much as possible to promote healing of the torn AF. The annular defect should be minimized. Patients with an annular defect greater than 6 mm showed higher recurrence and reoperation rates [12]. Thermal denaturation and annular collagen fibril shrinkage are believed to seal annular tears and stabilize the disc structure. Among various minimal invasive spinal interventions, neither extradiscal nor intradiscal applications alone seem adequate for successful treatment because of their limitations and risks. Thus, the simultaneous application of both procedures is required to achieve disc decompression and pain relief.

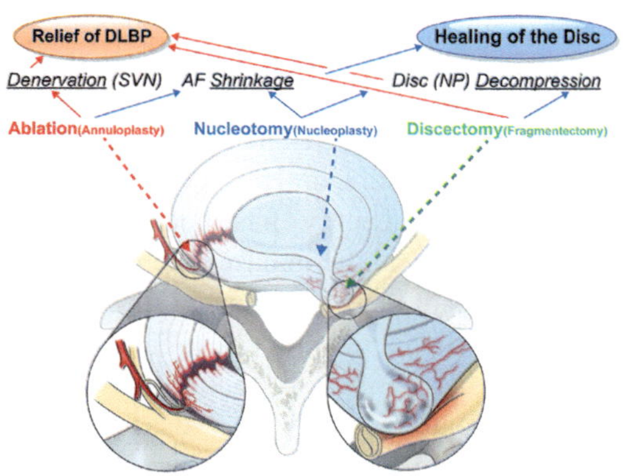

Fig. 9.2 Discogenic low back pain: goals, strategies, and treatment methods. SVN, sinuvertebral nerve; AF, annulus fibrosus; NP, nucleus pulposus

New techniques that combine transforaminal epiduroscopy with advanced laser technologies have recently become a focus of attention. Compared to the caudal approach, the transforaminal route offers many advantages, including more direct access to the ventral epidural space. Transforaminal epiduroscopy allows direct visualization of, and access to, spinal canal lesions and direct stimulation of the suspected pain generator with probes and a laser. Concordant pain provocation by direct stimulation can indicate the exact site of the pain generator. Furthermore, the degree of pain relief can be assessed during the treatment.

When thermal energy is used for discoplasty, the temperature must reach 45 °C to destroy the nociceptors and 60 °C to denaturize and shrink the collagen fibers [13]. The tissue is vaporized when heated rapidly to 100 °C or more [14]. Radiofrequency energy has been commonly used for intradiscal thermal treatment. However, there is a risk of thermal damage if heat diffuses to neighboring neural structures. The laser is an important therapeutic tool that is often used to ablate unwanted or abnormal tissue [15–17]. The pulsed holmium:yttrium-aluminum-garnet (Ho:YAG) laser emits light with a wavelength of 2100 nm and is the most commonly used laser for ablation therapy. This laser causes minimal damage to the adjacent normal soft tissue because of its low tissue penetration, and it is considered safe for surgical use. The end-firing Ho:YAG laser is used for PELAN procedures [18]. Unlike the conventional 1064-nm neodymium:yttrium-aluminum-garnet (Nd:YAG) laser that has deep tissue penetration, the new 1414-nm Nd:YAG laser has shallow penetration and can be used effectively and safely under the guidance of a spinal epiduroscope [19, 20] (Fig. 9.3). The 1414-nm Nd:YAG laser with side-firing fiber is used for TELA procedures. This instrument, under endoscopic guidance, seems suitable for the treatment of pain with a focal discogenic source, such as an annular tear or herniated nucleus pulposus (HNP). A study found that, compared to IDET, procedures using this laser within the AF caused a temperature increase within a relatively smaller radius [14]. Utilizing the appropriate laser and selecting the correct laser parameters can enhance the efficacy of discoplasty. Most spine procedures use a laser power setting of 5–20 W and an average of 1000–3000 J of energy delivered for ablation. However, this power setting is too high for laser discoplasty. The laser power level should be set to 2–6 W (200–300 mJ, 10–20 Hz) for denervation and coagulation and 6–12 W (300–600 mJ, 20 Hz) for vaporization and ablation [14].

This chapter describes discoplasty techniques that use a laser under epiduroscopic visualization and a transforaminal approach. Minimally invasive thermal annuloplasty and disc decompression can be achieved simultaneously. Currently, there are two approaches to endoscopic transforaminal discoplasty:

1. PELAN—for intradiscal applications only
2. TELA—for extradiscal applications with or without an intradiscal component

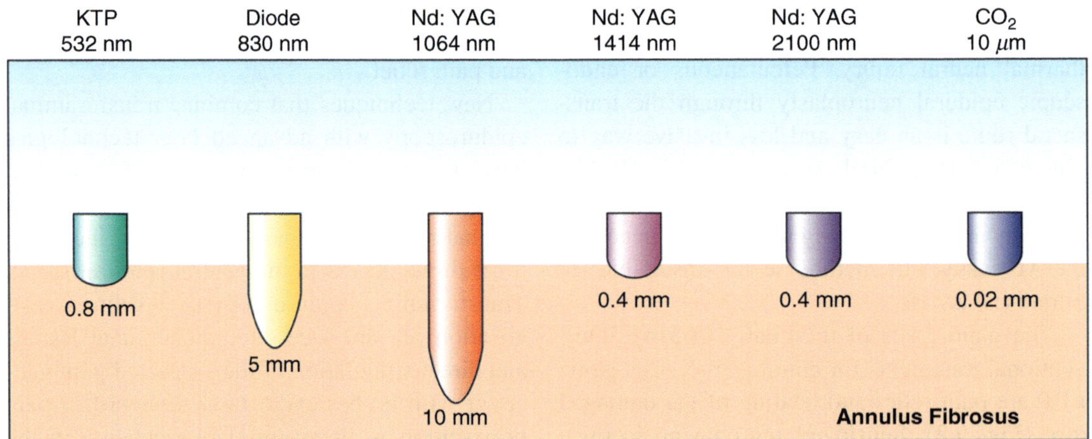

Fig. 9.3 Lasers used in spinal interventions: The 2100-nm holmium:yttrium-aluminum-garnet (Ho:YAG) laser used in percutaneous endoscopic lumbar annuloplasty and nucleoplasty and the 1414-nm neodymium:yttrium-aluminum-garnet (Nd:YAG) laser used in transforaminal epiduroscopic laser annuloplasty both have shallow tissue penetration. KTP, potassium-titanyl-phosphate; CO_2, carbon dioxide

9.3 Percutaneous Endoscopic Lumbar Annuloplasty and Nucleoplasty

PELAN is an intra-annular procedure that directly targets the granulation tissue in a torn AF. PELAN is performed with the patient in the prone position on a Wilson frame on a radiolucent operating table. The skin entry site is located approximately 10–13 cm from the midline and infiltrated with a local anesthetic. An 18-gauge spinal needle is inserted and advanced toward the foraminal zone AF. The needle tip is inserted just lateral to the medial pedicular line in the AP view and at the posterior vertebral line in the lateral view. The needle is inserted into the disc, and a discogram is obtained using a mixture of contrast medium and indigo carmine. The contrast medium serves to fill the annular fissure so that it can be seen in the AP and lateral fluoroscopic views, and the indigo carmine stains the nuclear materials in the annular fissure so that it can be endoscopically visualized.

A guidewire is then inserted through the needle into the AF. After a stab incision is made at the needle entry site, a working cannula is introduced over the guidewire and advanced into the posterior part of the AF. Under C-arm fluoroscopy, the cannula is placed in the AF as close as possible to the undersurface of the posterior longitudinal ligament. A flexible endoscopic catheter with a laser tip (LASE, Clarus Medical, Minneapolis, MN, US) is introduced through the cannula (Fig. 9.4). A Ho:YAG laser is used to

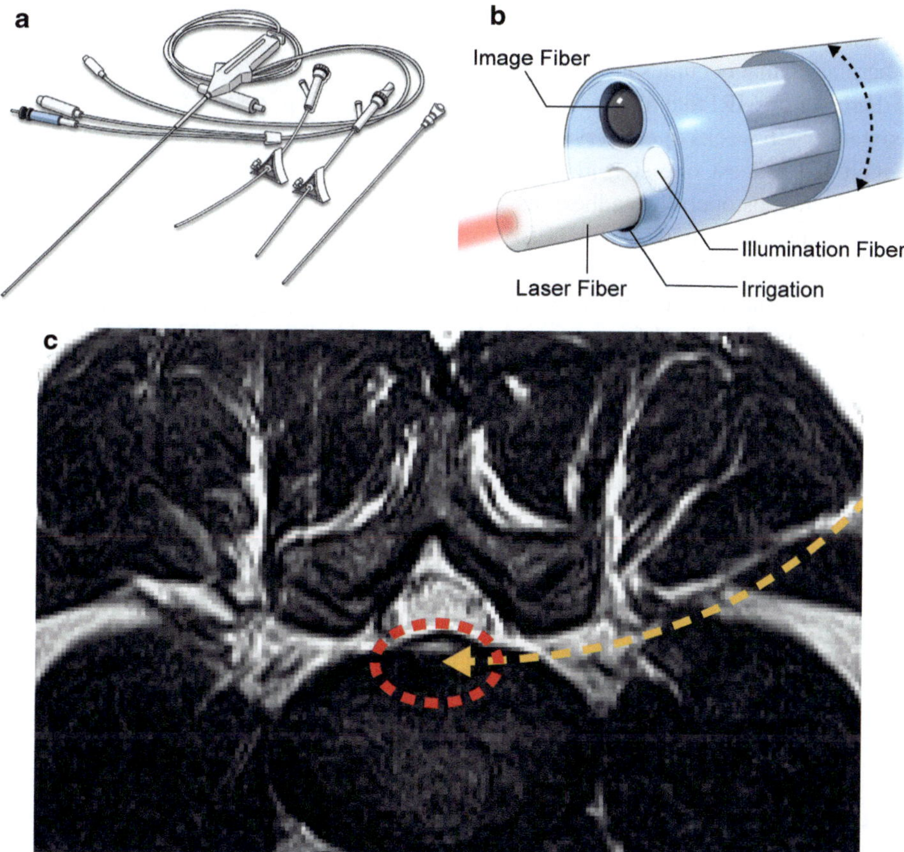

Fig. 9.4 A flexible endoscopic catheter (LASE, Clarus Medical, Minneapolis, MN, US) (**a**) equipped with a laser tip (**b**) is introduced through the cannula to target the granulation tissue in the torn annulus fibrosus (**c**) during percutaneous endoscopic lumbar annuloplasty and nucleoplasty

perform thermal ablation of the nuclear material and granulation tissue under direct endoscopic visualization. The laser power level is set to 0.5–1.2 J (10–20 Hz). Large nucleus pulposus fragments are released and removed using forceps. The procedure usually takes 30–45 min. The average total amount of laser energy delivered is 11,300 J. According to Lee et al., the success rate of annuloplasty performed using a laser as the heat source was 90% [18].

9.4 Transforaminal Epiduroscopic Laser Annuloplasty

9.4.1 Indications and Contraindications

Ideal candidates for TELA have discogenic LBP, with or without leg pain, secondary to an IAD and IVD herniation that occupies less than half of the canal diameter on MRI that has not responded to approximately 4–6 weeks of conservative therapy that included at least one steroid injection. Back pain due to postoperative adhesions and discal cysts can also be managed with TELA. In patients with discogenic LBP accompanied by mild to moderate neural foraminal stenosis, foraminoplasty using laser and forceps can help decompress the exiting nerve root. The SAP and transforaminal ligaments compressing the nerve root can be resected or vaporized. TELA contraindications are a neurological deficit, severe degenerative disc disease, severe neural foraminal stenosis, and segmental instability. The foraminal, central, and subarticular zones are easy to access [21] (Fig. 9.5). Access is difficult in cases of an HNP with distant, downward migration and L5–S1 lesions associated with a high iliac crest (Fig. 9.6).

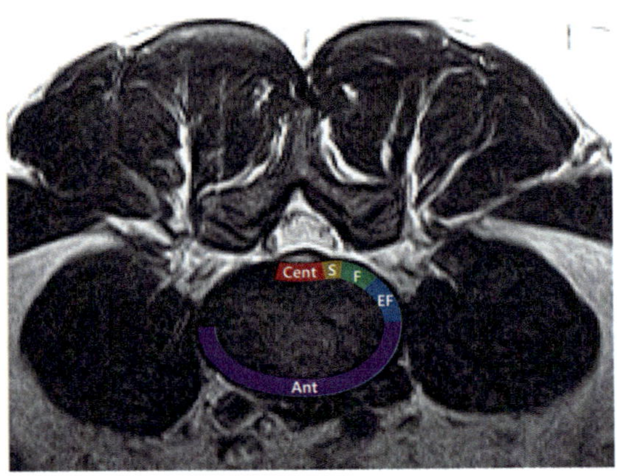

Fig. 9.5 Lumbar disc disease zones. Cent, central canal zone; S, subarticular (lateral recess) zone; F, foraminal zone; EF, extraforaminal (far lateral) zone; Ant, anterior zone. (Modified from Wiltse LL, Berger PE, McCulloch JA. A system for reporting the size and location of lesions in the spine. Spine. 1997;22:1534–1537)

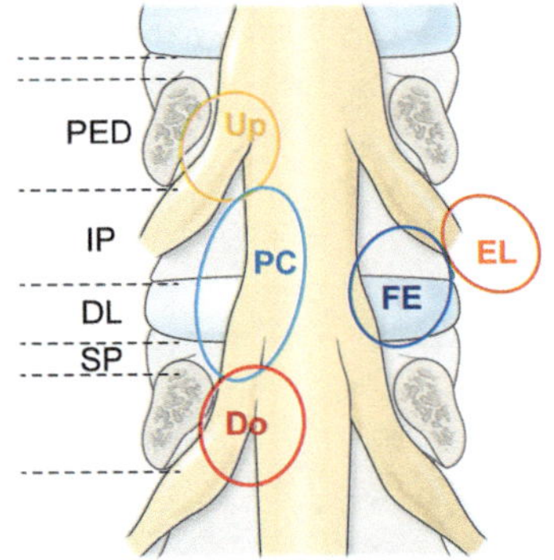

Fig. 9.6 Ease of access in transforaminal epiduroscopic laser annuloplasty (TELA). SP, suprapedicle level; PED, pedicle level; IP, infrapedicle level; DL, disc level; L, lumbar; T, thoracic; S, sacral; PC, paracentral (central and subarticular) zone; FE, foraminal and medial extraforaminal zone; EL, extreme lateral, lateral extraforaminal zone (lateral to exiting nerve root); Up, far upward-migrated HNP; Do, far downward-migrated HNP

9.4.2 Equipment and Instruments (Fig. 9.7)

1. Radiolucent operating table
2. C-arm fluoroscopic X-ray system
3. NeedleCam HD camera-monitor system (BioVision, Ilsan, ROK)
4. NeedleView CH endoscopy kit (Lutronic, Ilsan, ROK)
5. Accuplasti Laser (Lutronic)
6. Continuous gravity infusion irrigation system

9.4.2.1 NeedleView CH Endoscope Kit

The NeedleView CH is a disposable fiberoptic-based semirigid endoscope with a single working channel. The endoscope has a 160-mm working length with a 3.4-mm outer diameter, a 1.85-mm-diameter working channel, and a built-in 0.7-mm fiberoptic channel with 17,000-pixel resolution. The distal one-third of the endoscope can be bent to the desired angle to facilitate a transforaminal approach to the ventral epidural space (Fig. 9.8).

9.4.2.2 NeedleCam HD Camera-Monitor System

The NeedleCam HD system incorporates a light-emitting diode and a high-resolution camera in a single compact unit. The light source and video images are transmitted through a single cable (Fig. 9.9). The video output is connected to a high-definition display with a pixel resolution of 1920 × 1080.

9.4.2.3 Accuplasti Laser

The Accuplasti Laser is a pulsed Nd:YAG laser that delivers light with a wavelength of 1414-nm through a 550-μm laser fiber that is then transmitted through a 3-m fiber (Fig. 9.10).

9.4.2.4 Instruments for Introducing the Endoscope (Fig. 9.11)

1. 18-gauge × 152-mm spinal needle
2. 21-gauge × 400-mm spinal needle
3. 14-gauge × 127-mm Tuohy needle
4. 18-gauge × 152-mm Tuohy needle
5. 12-Fr cannula and 12-Fr dilator
6. 45-cm guidewire

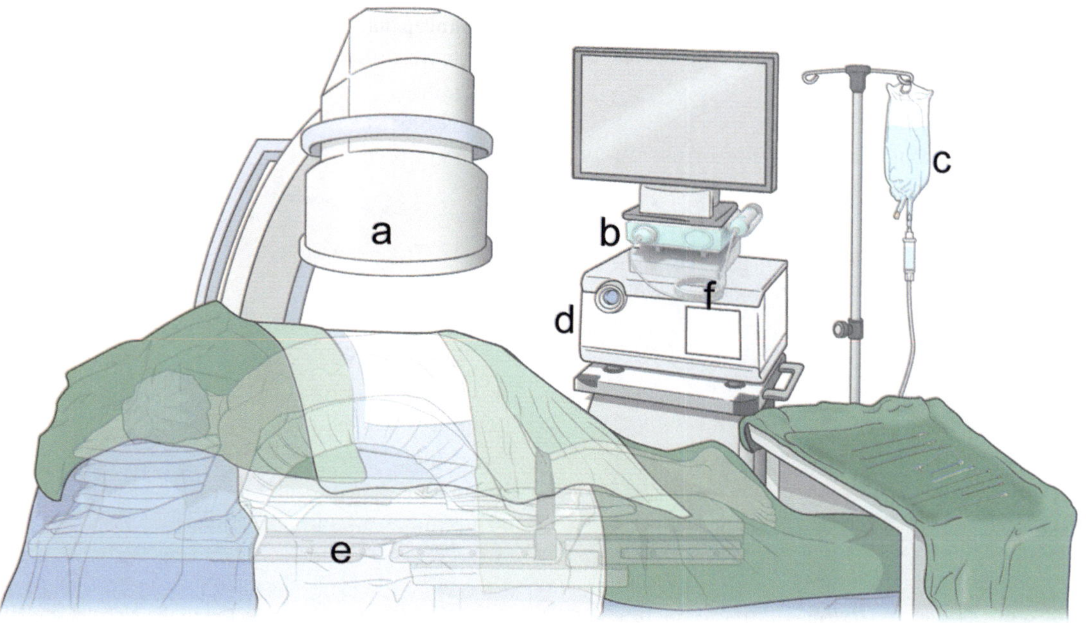

Fig. 9.7 Operating room setup, equipment, and instruments for transforaminal epiduroscopic laser annuloplasty: C-arm fluoroscopic X-ray system (**a**), NeedleCam HD camera-monitor system (BioVision, Ilsan, ROK) (**b**), continuous gravity-dependent infusion irrigation system (**c**), Accuplasti 1414-nm neodymium:yttrium-aluminum-garnet laser (Lutronic, Ilsan, ROK) (**d**), radiolucent operating table (**e**), and NeedleView CH endoscope optical fiber cable (Lutronic) (**f**) connected to the NeedleCam HD camera

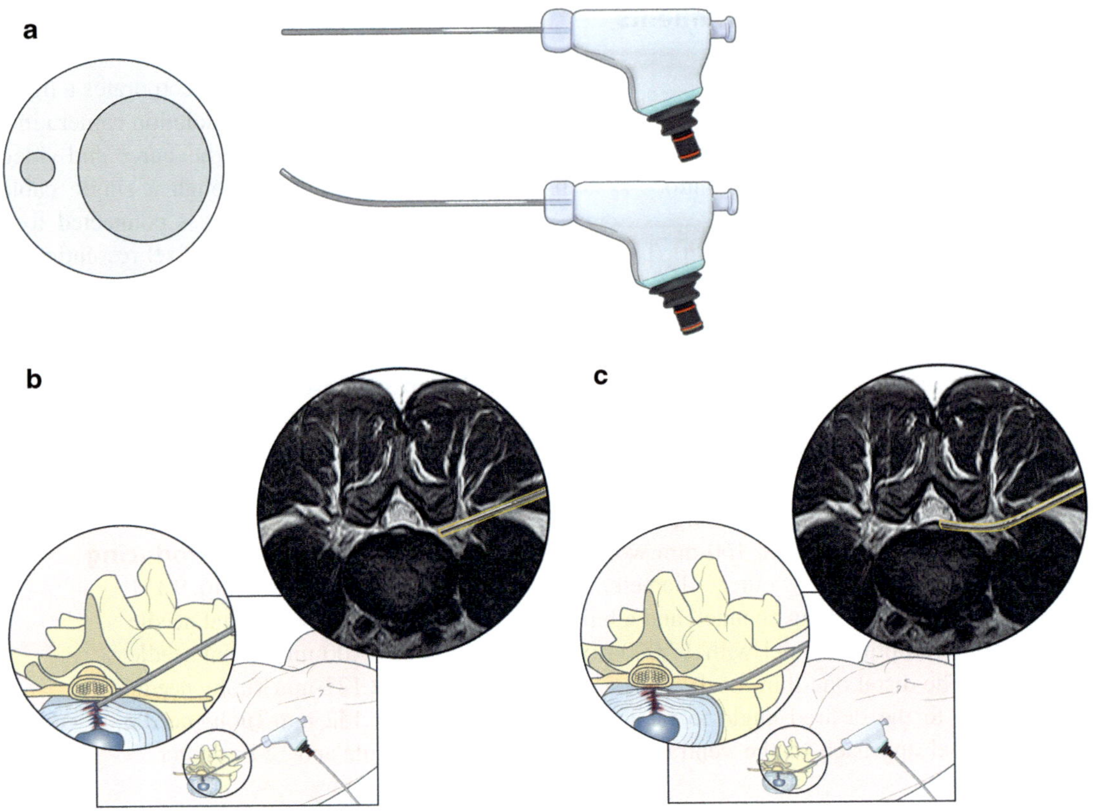

Fig. 9.8 NeedleView CH Endoscope (BioVision, Ilsan, ROK): Bent and straight NeedleView CH endoscopes (**a**): The straight scope is advanced toward the foraminal zone annulus fibrosus (**b**), and the bent scope is introduced into the ventral epidural space (**c**)

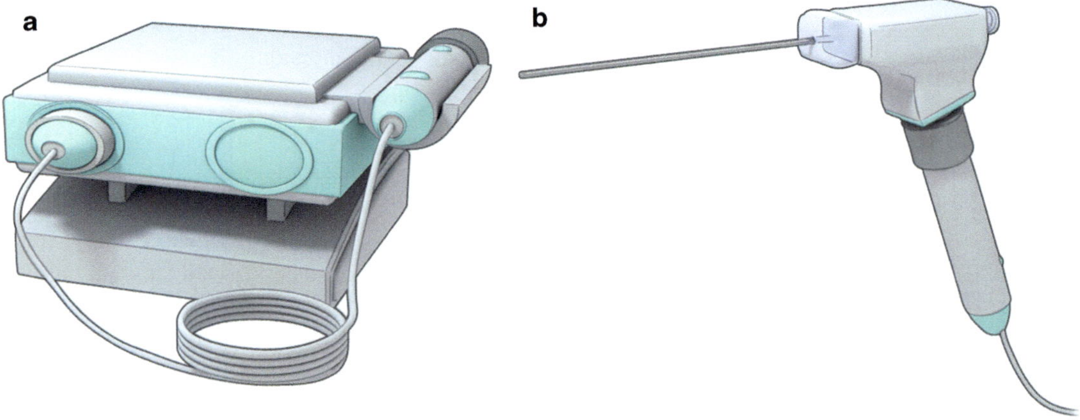

Fig. 9.9 NeedleCam HD camera (BioVision, Ilsan, ROK) (**a**), and NeedleView CH connected to the NeedleCam HD Camera handpiece (**b**)

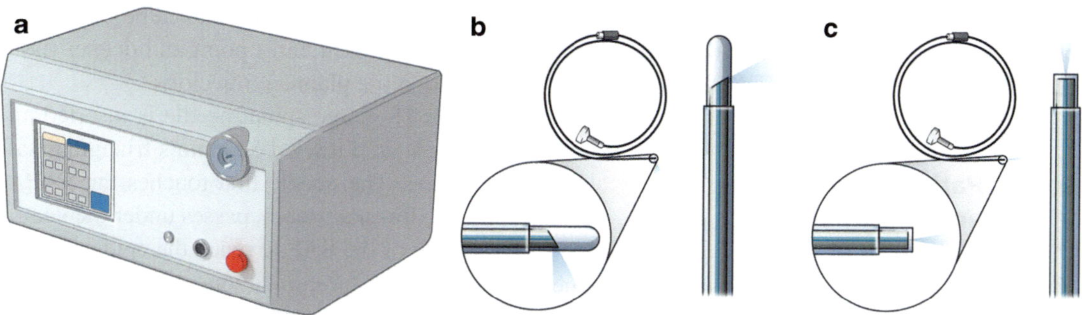

Fig. 9.10 Accuplasti Laser (**a**), side-firing laser fiber (**b**), and forward-firing laser fiber (**c**)

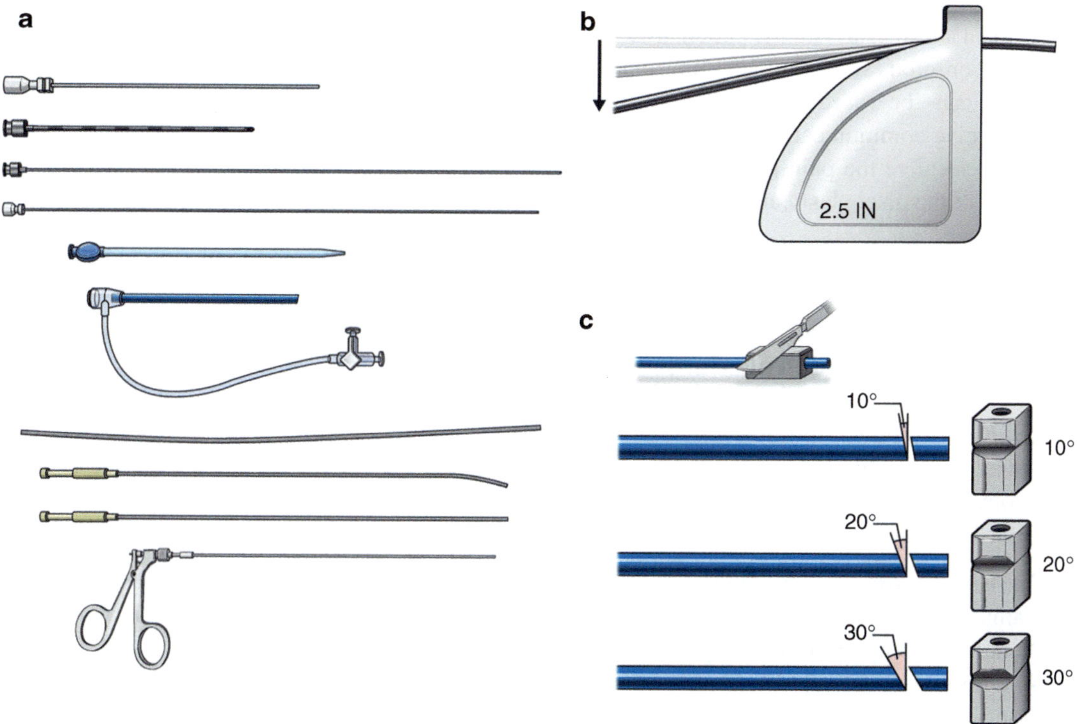

Fig. 9.11 Instruments for introducing the endoscope: 18-gauge × 152-mm spinal needle, 14-gauge × 127-mm Tuohy needle, 18-gauge × 152-mm Tuohy needle, 21-gauge × 400-mm spinal needle, 12-Fr cannula and 12-Fr dilator, 45-cm guidewire, probes, and 5-Fr × 300-mm endoscopic forceps (**a**), scope bender (**b**), and flexible dilator and cannula cutters (**c**)

7. Scope bender
8. Cannula cutter
9. 5-Fr × 300-mm grasping forceps

9.4.3 Preoperative Preparation and Operating Room Setup

Before beginning the procedure, axial MRI or CT images are used to determine the angle of approach and distance of the skin entry site from the midline for a trajectory to the neural foramen. The typical distance (for L3–L4–L5 levels) is 8–13 cm from the midline, and the approach angle is 20° to 30° from the horizon. A steeper angle of approach is recommended for upper lumbar levels (L1–L2–L3) and foraminal-extraforaminal lesions. An appropriate prophylactic antibiotic is used approximately 30 min before the procedure. Intraoperative monitoring, including electrocardiogram, blood pressure, and pulse oximetry, is initiated. The operating room setup for TELA is shown in Fig. 9.7.

9.4.4 Patient Positioning and Anesthesia

The patient is positioned prone on a Wilson frame on a radiolucent operating table and draped aseptically. The patient is maintained in a flexed position to increase the intervertebral foramen dimensions (Fig. 9.12). TELA is performed under local anesthesia with the patient awake and relaxed. Conscious sedation with midazolam and fentanyl can be used if needed. Effective intraoperative communication with the patient is critical to localize the pain generator and assess the effect of the discoplasty and for patient safety as well.

9.4.5 Recommended Steps of a Standard Procedure

Under Fluoroscopic Guidance

1. Spinal needle and guidewire insertion
2. Tuohy needle and guidewire advance
3. Dilator insertion and epidurography

Under Endoscopic Visualization

1. Cannula and epiduroscope insertion
2. Annular probing or discography or both
3. Annuloplasty, nucleoplasty, and discectomy, alone or combined

- Step 1: Insertion of Spinal Needle and Guidewire

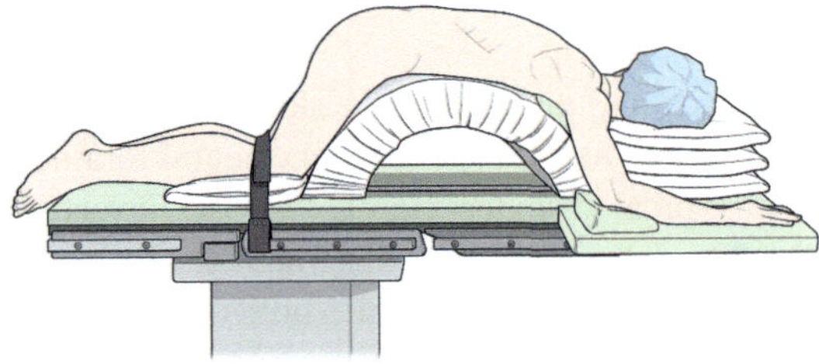

Fig. 9.12 The patient is positioned prone on a Wilson frame on a radiolucent operating table

  - Local anesthetic (1% lidocaine) is injected into the skin entry point and deeper tissue along the planned trajectory.
  - An 18-gauge spinal needle is inserted and navigated toward Kambin's triangular safe zone. The needle first touches the SAP of the lower vertebra, passes under the ventral side of the SAP to reach the epidural space near the foraminal zone AF [21], and then contacts the annular surface. The needle position is confirmed with AP and lateral fluoroscopy (Fig. 9.13).
  - The stylet is then removed, and a guidewire is passed into the epidural space at the lateral recess (subarticular zone). The epidural location of the guidewire is confirmed with AP and lateral fluoroscopic images.
- Step 2: Insertion of the Tuohy Needle and Guidewire Advancement
  - The spinal needle is removed, and a 14-gauge Tuohy needle is advanced over the guidewire into the epidural space, and the needle position is confirmed with fluoroscopy (Fig. 9.14).
  - The guidewire is then advanced within the ventral epidural space; forceful guidewire advancement can injure the AF, dura, or nerves.
  - The 14-gauge Tuohy needle is then removed, and the guidewire's location is confirmed with fluoroscopy.
- Step 3: Dilator Insertion and Epidurography
  - A 4-mm skin incision is made along the guidewire using a number 15 scalpel blade.
  - A plastic dilator is then passed gently over the guidewire. The ventral epidural location of the dilator is confirmed with AP and lateral fluoroscopy, and then the contrast agent is injected; filling defects and myelography findings should be investigated (Fig. 9.15).
- Step 4: Cannula and Epiduroscope Insertion
  - The 12-Fr dilator and the 12-Fr cannula are inserted together over the guidewire, and the dilator is then removed.
  - The NeedleView CH endoscope is inserted through the cannula and advanced toward the annular surface at the foraminal zone.

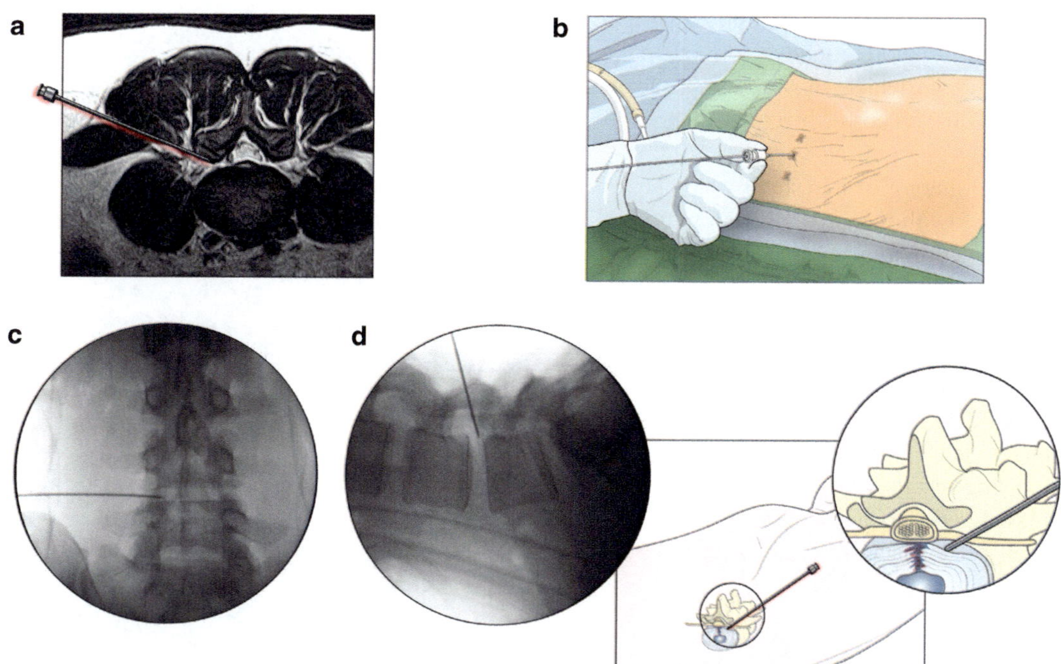

Fig. 9.13 Step 1: Insertion of the spinal needle and guidewire: An 18-gauge spinal needle is inserted into the epidural space at the lateral recess (subarticular zone) (**a**), and a guidewire is passed through the needle (**b**). The needle position is confirmed with anteroposterior (**c**) and lateral (**d**) fluoroscopy

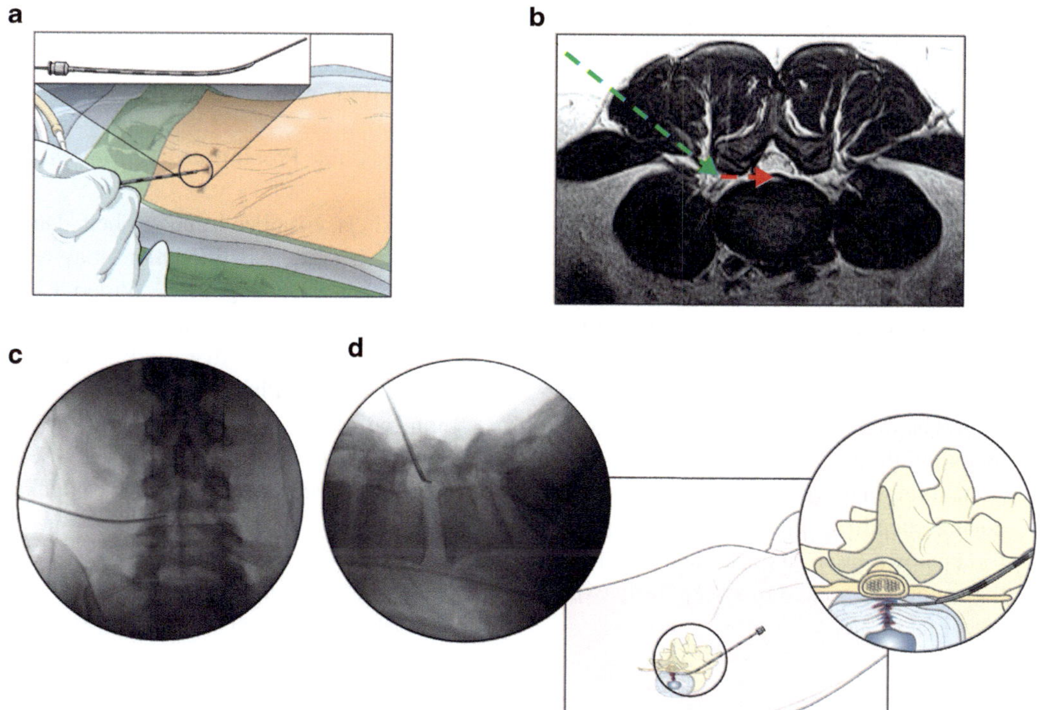

Fig. 9.14 Step 2: Insertion of a Tuohy needle and guidewire advancement: A 14-gauge Tuohy needle is passed over the guidewire into the epidural space (**a**); the guidewire is then advanced in the ventral epidural space (**b**). The needle and guidewire positions are confirmed with anteroposterior (**c**) and lateral (**d**) fluoroscopy

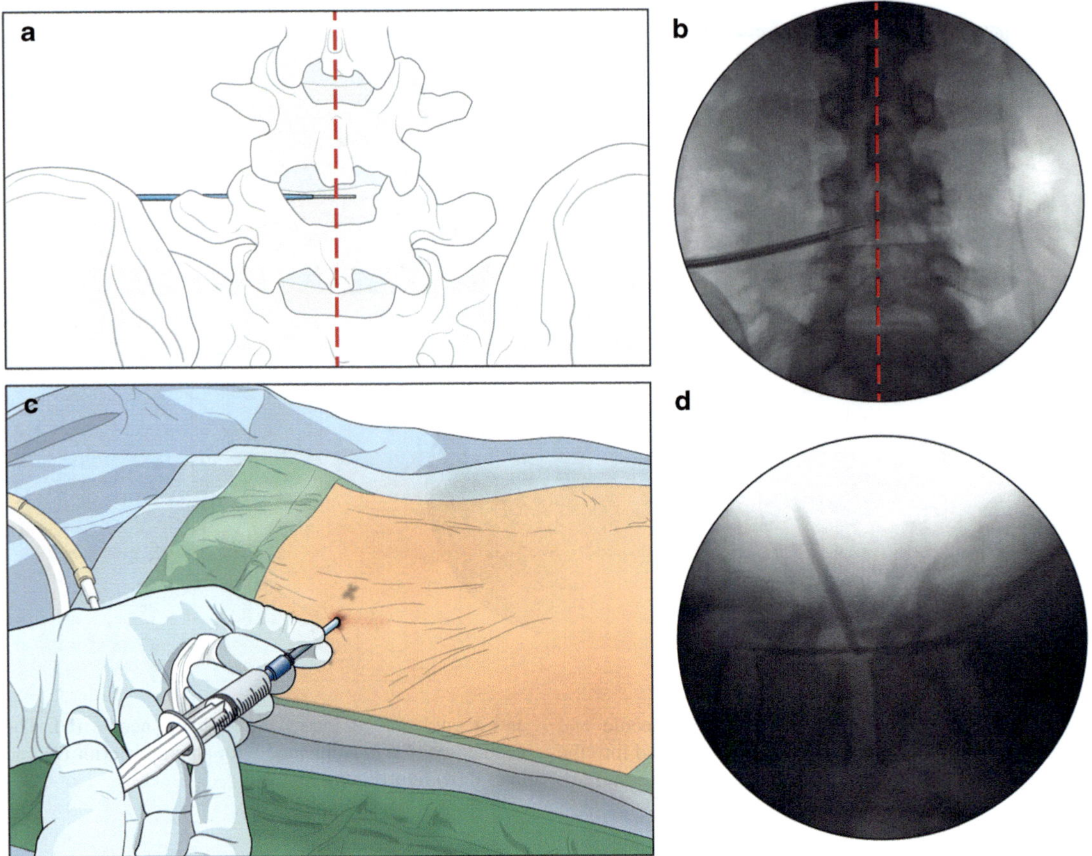

Fig. 9.15 Step 3: Dilator insertion and epidurography: A plastic dilator is passed over the guidewire and advanced into the ventral epidural space (**a**, **b**), and contrast agent is injected through the dilator (**c**, **d**)

  - Irrigation is started before the endoscope is manipulated. The bag of irrigation fluid (0.9% normal saline) is suspended on an IV stand at a suitable height above the patient (Fig. 9.7). Normally, a height of 30 to 50 cm is recommended for patient safety. If bleeding obstructs the operator's view of the surgical field, the irrigation pressure should be increased by raising the height of irrigation fluid.
  - Transforaminal ligaments encountered during sheath insertion are resected with forceps or a laser, and the beveled end of the cannula is rotated to sweep away extradiscal fat tissue.

- Step 5: Annular Probing and Chromodiscography
  - The AF is visualized and probed. During palpation of the AF, the patient may report concordant LBP (Fig. 9.16) (Video 9.1).
  - Chromodiscography can be performed with a mixture of dye (indigo carmine, Korea United Pharm, Seoul, ROK) and non-iodinated contrast (iohexol [Omnipaque, GE Healthcare Korea, Seoul, ROK]); concordant pain or dye leakage may occur.
  - Radicular pain or neurophysiological electromyography monitoring findings may indicate pressure on the nerve root, which

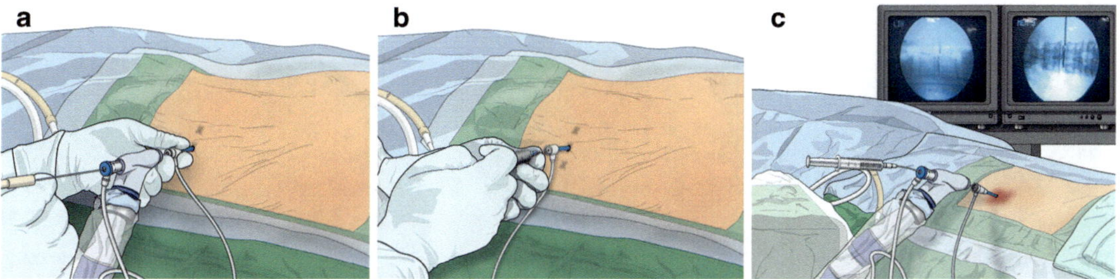

Fig. 9.16 Step 5: Annular probing and chromodiscography: localization of the pain generator using an annular probing technique (**a**) and chromodiscography (**b**); contrast leakage may occur (**c**)

should prompt the operator to redirect the device.

- Step 6: Annuloplasty, Nucleoplasty, and Fragmentectomy (Discectomy)
  - The NeedleView endoscope is bent to the appropriate angle and inserted through the neural foramen, followed by endoscopic visualization of the ventral epidural anatomy.
  - Findings may include a torn, reddish, hyperemic, or indigo carmine-stained AF, dye leakage, HNP, or concordant pain with probing of the torn AF (Fig. 9.17).
  - The Accuplasti Laser is then introduced through the working channel of the NeedleView CH scope into the epidural space, and the laser parameters are selected.
  - The appropriate setting for hemostasis, thermal denervation, and shrinkage of the torn AF is 150–300 mJ at 10–20 Hz and less than 6 W. A laser power of 6–12 W is recommended for vaporization; higher power should be used cautiously and only with clear visualization and continuous saline irrigation (Table 9.1).
  - The AF can be punctured with a sharpened wire, forward-firing laser, or endoscopic forceps if needed.
  - The operator should not attempt to vaporize the whole nuclear fragment. Endoscopic forceps can also be used to remove free fragments.
  - Low-power lasering is used to shrink the decompressed the AF and annular defects.

9.4.6 Discoplasty Variations

The operator should select the appropriate TELA variation based on the degree of annular tearing and nucleus pulposus herniation (Fig. 9.18):

1. Annuloplasty (TELA) is an extradiscal procedure that should only be used when intradiscal removal is not required. The AF is not punctured, and laser irradiation is only applied to its torn outer surface. When a disc sequestrum is identified, but chromodiscography shows no leakage, an annular puncture is not required (Fig. 9.19). The sensitized sinuvertebral nerves around the annular tear in outer AF can be directly denervated with lasering under epiduroscopic visualization (Fig. 9.17). Sealing of the annular tear or shrinkage of the HIZ can be seen in follow-up MRI after TELA (Fig. 9.19).
2. Annulo-nucleoplasty (TELAN) is TELA with the addition of annular puncture and removal of herniated or interposed nucleus pulposus material from the annular fissure. It is a combined intradiscal and extradiscal procedure (Video 9.2).
3. Discectomy (fragmentectomy) and annuloplasty (TELDA) are used for the removal of contained and non-contained nucleus pulposus fragments. If a sequestered HNP is present, then fragmentectomy is followed by either annuloplasty or annulo-nucleoplasty.
4. Foraminoplasty (TELF) is performed when foraminal stenosis is accompanied by a primary lesion such as an HNP or annular tear (Video 9.3).

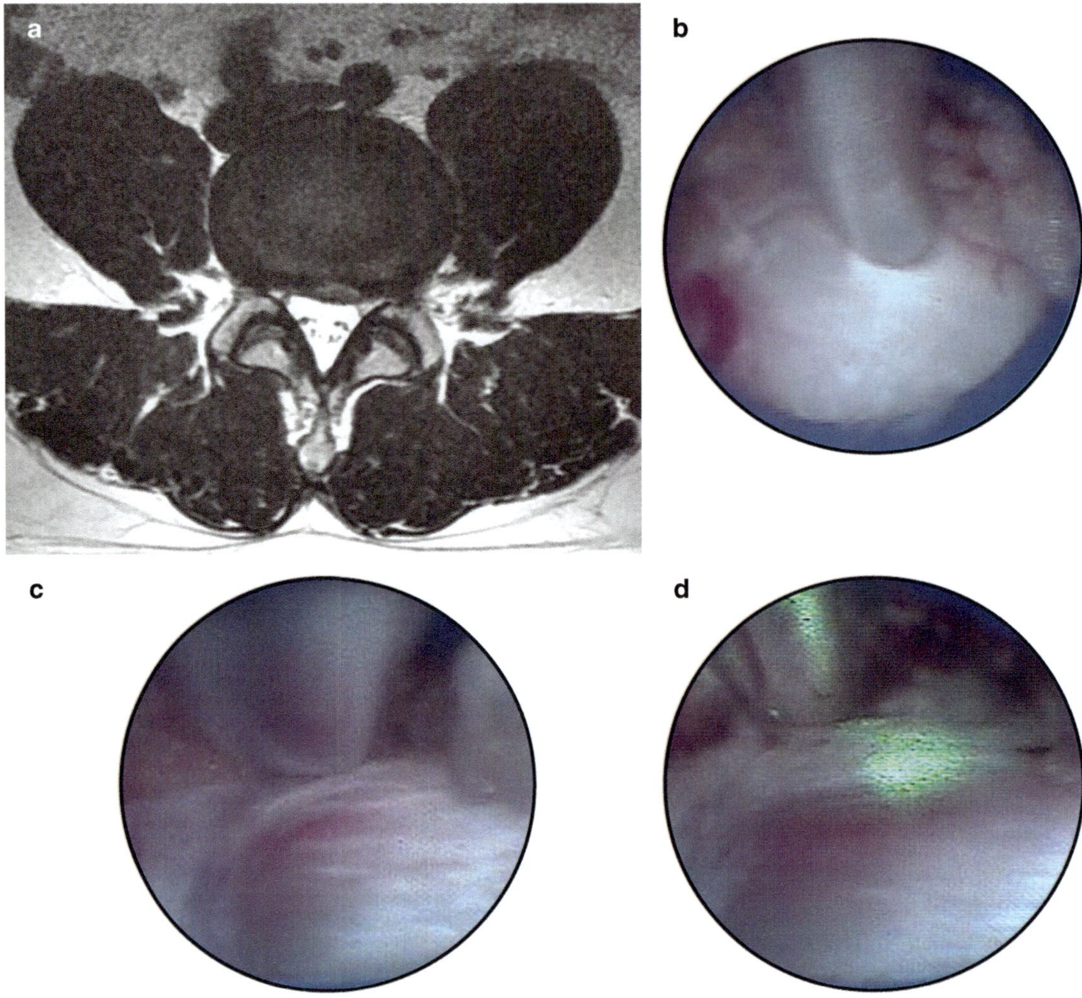

Fig. 9.17 Localization of the pain generator using an annular probing technique and laser annuloplasty: Preoperative axial T2-weighted magnetic resonance imaging shows a high-intensity zone at the central posterior annulus fibrosus (**a**). Pain is not provoked with annular probing of an intact annulus fibrosus (**b**). Concordant back pain is provoked by probe stimulation of the inflamed hyperemic annulus fibrosus (**c**). Annuloplasty with side-firing 1414-nm neodymium:yttrium-aluminum-garnet laser (**d**)

Table 9.1 Power settings for the 1414-nm neodymium:yttrium-aluminum-garnet laser

Mode	Tissues	Pulse energy (mJ)	Frequency (Hz)
Stimulation	Annulus Fibrosus	100–150	10
Shrinkage and denervation	Blood vessels	150–250	15–20
	Nucleus pulposus	150–250	15–20
	Annulus fibrosus	200–300	15–20
Vaporization	Epidural fat	300–400	20
	Nucleus pulposus	300–400	20
	Annulus fibrosus	400–500	20
	Transforaminal ligaments	400–500	20
	Bone (spur, superior articular process)	500–600	20

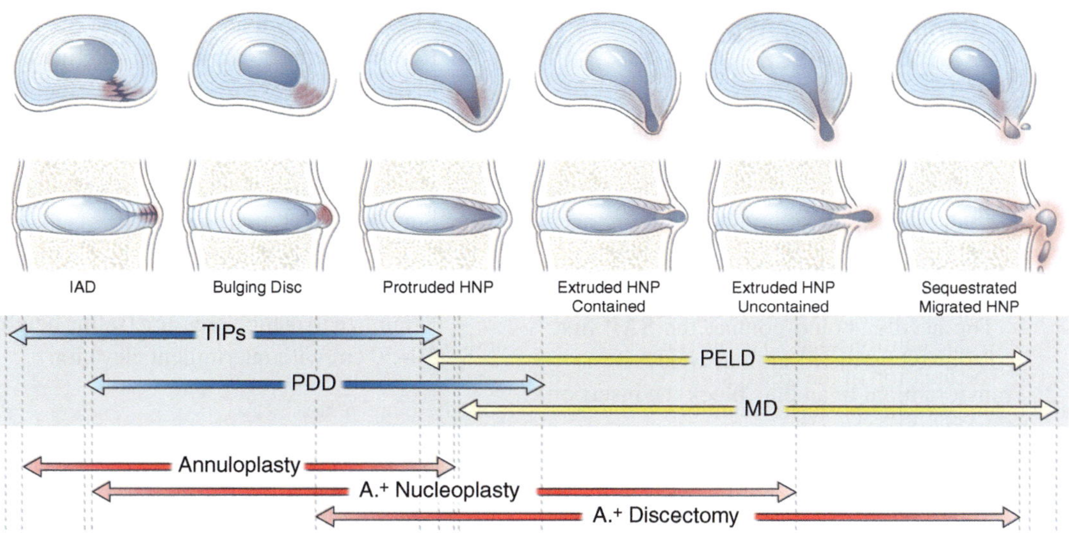

Fig. 9.18 The degree of annular tearing and nucleus pulposus herniation determine the appropriate procedure: annuloplasty (TELA), annulo-nucleoplasty (TELAN), or discectomy (fragmentectomy), and annuloplasty (TELDA). IAD, internal annular disruption; HNP, herniated nucleus pulposus; TIPs, thermal intradiscal procedures; PDD, percutaneous disc decompression; PELD, percutaneous endoscopic lumbar discectomy; MD, microscopic discectomy; A., annuloplasty

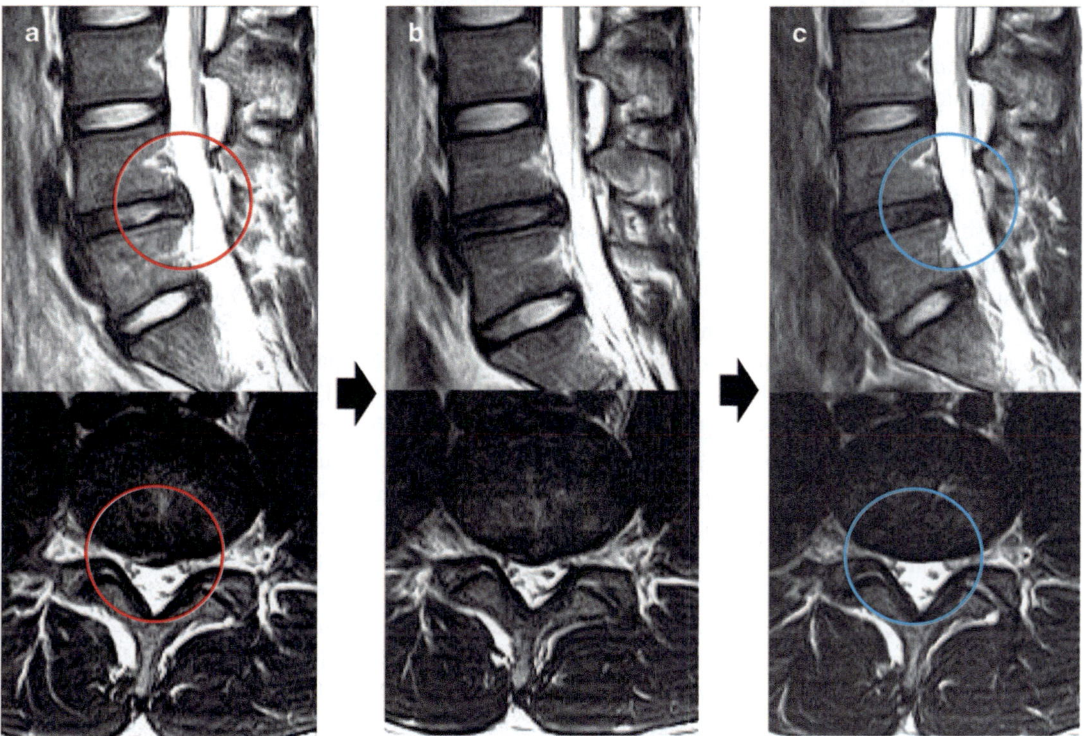

Fig. 9.19 Shrinkage of annular tear after transforaminal epiduroscopic laser annuloplasty: Preoperative magnetic resonance imaging (MRI) in a 22-year-old man shows a high intensity zone (HIZ) at the L4–L5 posterior annulus fibrosus (**a**). An immediate postoperative MRI study after transforaminal epiduroscopic laser annuloplasty shows decreased HIZ size (**b**). A postoperative MRI performed 2 years later shows no HIZ (**c**)

9.4.7 Complications: Avoidance and Management

1. Injury of the exiting nerve root or abdominal contents during needle insertion
   - The skin entry point should be less than 13 cm lateral to the midline.
   - The angle of approach should be more than 20°.
   - The needle should contact the SAP first, followed by the foraminal zone AF.
2. Transforaminal ligaments block the insertion of the working sheath.
   - Resect or vaporize obstructing transforaminal ligaments before inserting the working cannula.
3. Neural foramen stenosis
   - The SAP and foraminal ligaments can be partially removed with laser or forceps.
4. Annular damage
   - Insert instruments gently.
   - Decrease the laser power when performing annuloplasty.
   - Apply continuous saline irrigation while lasering.
   - Create the smallest possible annular puncture with a straight laser (1 mm), sharpened wire, or grasping forceps (5 Fr).
5. Infection
   - Use single-use instruments, aseptic technique, and prophylactic antibiotics.
6. Instrument damage
   - Handle the instruments with care.
   - Operate under clear visualization.
7. Bleeding
   - Apply laser coagulation and cotton packing and allow time for hemostasis.
   - Temporarily increase the irrigation pressure by raising the height of the irrigation fluid container.
8. Dural or neural injury by instrumentation or thermal injury by laser
   - An awake procedure under local or epidural anesthesia is mandatory.
   - Select an adequate angle of trajectory and bend the scope sufficiently.
   - Lasering should be performed at low power under clear visualization.
9. Incomplete removal and recurrence of HNP
   - Remove all loose intradiscal fragments.
   - Minimize the existing annular defect and avoid iatrogenic annular injuries.
10. Headache, neck pain, and increased ICP
    - Keep the patient's head elevated throughout the procedure to avoid a headache.
    - If a headache occurs, raise the patient's head.
    - Minimize irrigation pressure (saline height, 30–50 cm with intermittent elevation)

9.5 Conclusions

Ji et al. reported that TELA is superior to a selective transforaminal epidural block procedure for the treatment of single-level disc disease in decreasing pain and improving the quality of life over 1 year [22]. Kim et al. showed that TELA could provide immediate pain relief and reported a 96.1% success rate [23]. Park and Lee compared the benefits and complications after disc decompression by endoscopic epidural laser decompression and TELA and found that the procedures provided similar outcomes [24]. In another study, Park et al. compared the pain scores and disability indices of patients who underwent intradiscal radiofrequency annuloplasty (IDRA) or transforaminal laser annuloplasty and reported that TELA might be superior to IDRA in patients with discogenic LBP [25].

Both TELA and PELAN are valid treatment options for symptomatic lumbar spine annular tears and HNP. TELA allows annular probing and chromodiscography under visual guidance, and these techniques are particularly helpful for pain generator localization. The diagnosis of annulogenic, discogenic LBP is strongly supported by the occurrence of concordant pain with annular stimulation before and instant pain relief after laser irradiation.

Epiduroscopic laser discoplasty allows denervation as well as disc sealing, theoretically, providing pain relief as well as promoting disc healing. Endoscopic techniques and laser technology both continue to evolve in the management of various spinal pathologies.

References

1. DePalma MJ, Ketchum JM, Saullo T. What is the source of chronic low back pain and does age play a role? Pain Med. 2011;12:224–33.
2. Peng BG. Pathophysiology, diagnosis, and treatment of discogenic low back pain. World J Orthop. 2013;4:42–52.
3. Yoshizawa H, O'Brien JP, Smith WT, Trumper M. The neuropathology of intervertebral discs removed for low-back pain. J Pathol. 1980;132:95–104.
4. Crock HV. A reappraisal of intervertebral disc lesions. Med J Aust. 1970;1:983–9.
5. Jha SC, Higashino K, Sakai T, Takata Y, Abe M, Yamashita K, et al. Clinical significance of high intensity zone for discogenic low back pain: a review. J Med Investig. 2016;63:1–7.
6. Sachs BL, Vanharanta H, Spivey MA, Guyer RD, Videman T, Rashbaum RF, et al. Dallas discogram description. A new classification of CT/discography in low-back disorders. Spine (Phila Pa 1976). 1987;12:287–94.
7. Kuslich SD, Ulstrom CL, Michael CJ. The tissue origin of low back pain and sciatica: a report of pain response to tissue stimulation during operations on the lumbar spine using local anesthesia. Orthop Clin North Am. 1991;22:181–7.
8. Singh K, Ledet E, Carl A. Intradiscal therapy: a review of current treatment modalities. Spine (Phila Pa 1976). 2005;30(17 Suppl):S20–6.
9. Bosscher HA, Heavner JE. Diagnosis of the vertebral level from which low back or leg pain originates. A comparison of clinical evaluation, MRI and epiduroscopy. Pain Pract. 2012;12:506–12.
10. Bosscher HA, Heavner JE. Lumbosacral epiduroscopy findings predict treatment outcome. Pain Pract. 2014;14:506–14.
11. Lee GW, Jang SJ, Kim JD. The efficacy of epiduroscopic neural decompression with Ho:YAG laser ablation in lumbar spinal stenosis. Eur J Orthop Surg Traumatol. 2014;24(Suppl 1):S231–7.
12. Miller LE, McGirt MJ, Garfin SR, Bono CM. Association of annular defect width after lumbar discectomy with risk of symptom recurrence and reoperation: systematic review and meta-analysis of comparative studies. Spine (Phila Pa 1976). 2018;43:E308–15.
13. Freeman BJ, Walters RM, Moore RJ, Fraser RD. Does intradiscal electrothermal therapy denervate and repair experimentally induced posterolateral annular tears in an animal model? Spine (Phila Pa 1976). 2003;28:2602–8.
14. Lee MH, Kim IS, Hong JT, Sung JH, Lee SW, Kim DH. Temperature distributions of the lumbar intervertebral disc during laser annuloplasty: a cadaveric study. J Korean Neurosurg Soc. 2016;59:559–63.
15. Choy DS, Case RB, Fielding W, Hughes J, Liebler W, Ascher P. Percutaneous laser nucleolysis of lumbar disks. N Engl J Med. 1987;317:771–2.
16. Choy DS, Ascher PW, Ranu HS, Saddekni S, Alkaitis D, Liebler W, et al. Percutaneous laser disc decompression: a new therapeutic modality. Spine (Phila Pa 1976). 1992;17:949–56.
17. Gangi A, Dietemann JL, Ide C, Brunner P, Klinkert A, Warter JM. Percutaneous laser disk decompression under CT and fluoroscopic guidance: indications, technique, and clinical experience. Radiographics. 1996;16:89–96.
18. Lee SH, Kang HS. Percutaneous endoscopic laser annuloplasty for discogenic low back pain. World Neurosurg. 2010;73:198–206; discussion e33.
19. Jayasree RS, Gupta AK, Bodhey NK, Mohanty M. Effect of 980-nm diode laser and 1064-nm Nd:YAG laser on the intervertebral disc--in vitro and in vivo studies. Photomed Laser Surg. 2009;27:547–52.
20. Moon BJ, Lee HY, Kim KN, Yi S, Ha Y, Yoon DH, et al. Experimental evaluation of percutaneous lumbar laser disc decompression using a 1414 nm Nd:YAG laser. Pain Physician. 2015;18:E1091–9.
21. Wiltse LL, Berger PE, McCulloch JA. A system for reporting the size and location of lesions in the spine. Spine. 1997;22:1534–7.
22. Ji GY, Lee J, Lee SW, Cho BY, Ha DW, Park YM, et al. Safety and effectiveness of transforaminal epiduroscopic laser ablation in single level disc disease: a case-control study. Pain Physician. 2018;21:E643–50.
23. Kim HS, Paudel B, Chung SK, Jang JS, Oh SH, Jang IT. Transforaminal epiduroscopic laser ablation of sinuvertebral nerve in patients with chronic diskogenic back pain: technical note and preliminary result. J Neurol Surg A Cent Eur Neurosurg. 2017;78:529–34.
24. Park CH, Lee SH. Endoscopic epidural laser decompression versus transforaminal epiduroscopic laser annuloplasty for lumbar disc herniation: a prospective, randomized trial. Pain Physician. 2017;20:663–70.
25. Park CH, Lee KK, Lee SH. Efficacy of transforaminal laser annuloplasty versus intradiscal radiofrequency annuloplasty for discogenic low back pain. Korean J Pain. 2019;32:113–9.

Trans-sacral Discoplasty with Epiduroscopy

10

Sang Hyuk Park

10.1 Introduction

The epidural space is a potential space that contains semi-liquid fat, lymphatics, arteries, loose areolar connective tissue, the spinal nerve roots, and an extensive venous plexus. This space lies between the dura and the IVDs, bones, and ligaments of the spinal canal. Pain is provoked by epidural space defects that cause nerve root stimulation, such as ruptured IVDs and epidural adhesions [1–4]. There are two approaches to the epidural space: anterior and posterior. Anatomically, the spinal nerve originates from the ventral part of the thecal sac, and the IVD is in the same space. Therefore, the ventral epidural space is an important site of spinal pain treatment [5].

In 1931, Burman performed the first vertebral epiduroscopy using a rigid arthroscopic system in a cadaver [6]. Pool performed the first myeloscopic approach to the spine in anesthetized patients in 1937 and illustrated the endoscopic evaluation results of 400 patients with medical drawings in 1942 [7]. Leu introduced the sacral approach with epidural intraductal endoscopy [8].

Endoscopic equipment has substantially improved with the development of fiber optic light source technology. Intra- and extradural endoscopy methods were developed by Ooi between 1960 and 1970, and he added a fiber optic light source to the system to allow intraoperative photography [9]. Saberski and Kitahata developed the flexible fiberoptic endoscope and light systems in 1991 [10, 11]. In 1996, the United States Food and Drug Administration approved the use of epiduroscopy for visualization of the epidural space.

Although epiduroscopic procedures have been used for many years and sufficient evidence has accumulated to demonstrate the efficacy of spinal pain treatment, until recently, it was not possible to remove material from the epidural space using epiduroscopy, and some clinicians questioned whether it would be. However, a clinical trial of laser nerve decompression by evaporating the ruptured nucleus pulposus and ablating adhesive soft tissue demonstrated favorable results. Epiduroscopy with laser ablation has gradually become a widely used and effective treatment for spinal pain [12, 13].

10.2 Indications

1. An insufficient response to conservative treatment provided for at least 6 months.
2. Back pain related to an annular tear, i.e., discogenic back pain.

S. H. Park (✉)
Yonsei Barowalk Clinic, Anyang-si, Republic of Korea

S.-H. Lee (ed.), *Minimally Invasive Spine Interventions*,
https://doi.org/10.1007/978-981-16-9547-6_10

3. Massive lumbar disc herniation or one with proximally or distally sequestered fragments.
4. Root irritation secondary to epidural adhesions.
5. Discal cyst.
6. FBSS.
7. Patients who cannot undergo surgery because of age or general medical condition.

10.3 Contraindications

1. Moderate to severe stenosis.
2. Calcified disc lesions.
3. A sacral shape such as steep angle or caudal canal stenosis that is unsuitable for an approach to the epidural space.
4. A closed sacral hiatus.
5. Systemic or local infection.
6. Lumbar instability, lumbar spondylolisthesis, or both.
7. Cauda equina syndrome.
8. Systemic medical diseases including a bleeding tendency and coagulopathies.

10.4 Technical Aspects of Epiduroscopy

10.4.1 Instruments

10.4.1.1 Epidural Dual Channel Catheter

This bidirectional steerable catheter has two working channels (lumens) that are 30 cm long and have an outer diameter of 3 mm. The catheter is a little stiff, so it can be manipulated while maintaining a position such that the upper and lower working channels are not distorted during the procedure.

Both working channels have a diameter of 1.3 mm. The upper channel is for a high-resolution fiber optic camera, and the lower channel is for a laser fiber and epiduroscopic pituitary grasping forceps that can perform mechanical decompression by removing tissues. The catheter also has a dual infusion port for water irrigation, drainage, and drug injection (Fig. 10.1).

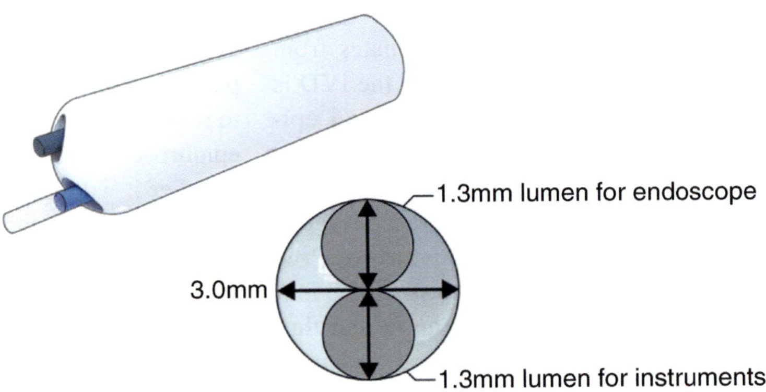

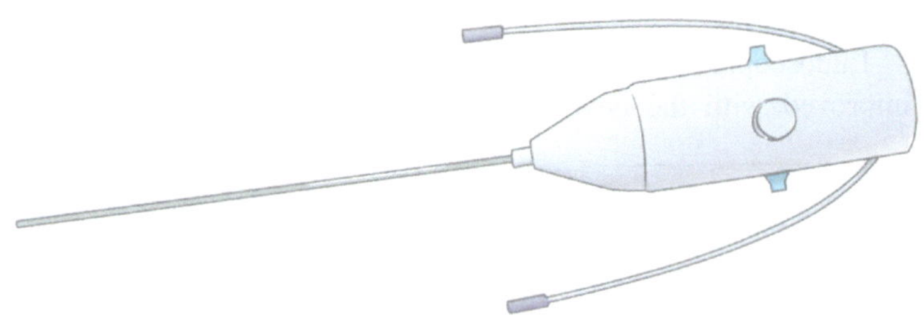

Fig. 10.1 An epidural dual-channel catheter

10.4.1.2 Flexible Fiber Optic Epiduroscope

The flexible fiber optic epiduroscope we use is 1.3 mm in outer diameter and 125 cm long. It enters through the top channel of the catheter. It has approximately 40× magnification, 17,000 pixels, and a 0-degree angle of view and is compatible with a universal camera system (Fig. 10.2).

10.4.1.3 Laser System

The VersaPulse P20 laser system (Lumenis Medical Solutions, Yokneam, Israel) with a Ho:YAG laser is used for treatment. The Ho:YAG laser has a high affinity for water at a wavelength of 2.1 μm and a relatively shallow penetration depth of <0.4 mm in disc tissue. Other benefits include minimal heat generation, low tissue permeability, good gasification, and minimal damage to surrounding tissues such as the dura or nerve roots (Fig. 10.3).

10.4.2 Surgical Approach and Technical Notes

Step 1. Preparation

- Preoperative preparation.
  - It is essential to confirm the indications for trans-sacral discoplasty by correlating the patient's symptoms with their MRI findings.
  - It is important to confirm the presence of symptoms using neurological examinations, such as the straight leg raise test.
  - Preoperatively, the dural sac (identified on MRI) and the lumbosacral angle must be measured.
  - A precise medication history, including anticoagulant therapy, should be recorded.
- Patient preparation.
  - Trans-sacral discoplasty is performed with the patient in the prone position on a radiolucent table in a sterile operating room.

Step 2. Patient in a Prone Position on a Wilson Frame

- Physiological parameters such as blood pressure, pulse rate, and pulse oximetry are monitored in preparation for an emergency.
- Pressure points are relieved using footpads, head gel, and arm supports, and a Wilson frame can be used to minimize lumbar lordosis and maximize lumbar flexion; the reduction of lumbosacral lordosis allows an easy approach to the target (Fig. 10.4).

Step 3. Sacral Hiatus Skin Incision

- The skin is prepped and draped to ensure asepsis, and 1% lidocaine is administered at the sacral hiatus.
- A 0.5 cm longitudinal skin incision is made in the sacral hiatus (Fig. 10.5).
- A trocar needle is used to puncture the sacrococcygeal ligament in the sacral hiatus.

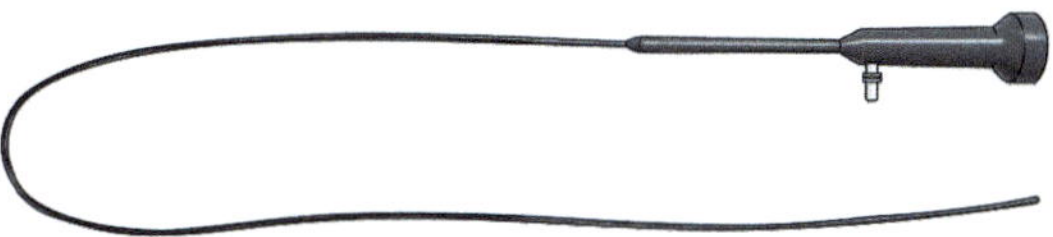

Fig. 10.2 A flexible fiber optic epiduroscope

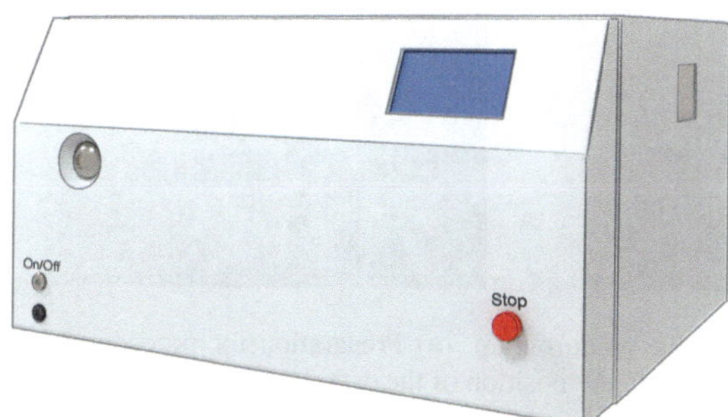

Fig. 10.3 The laser system

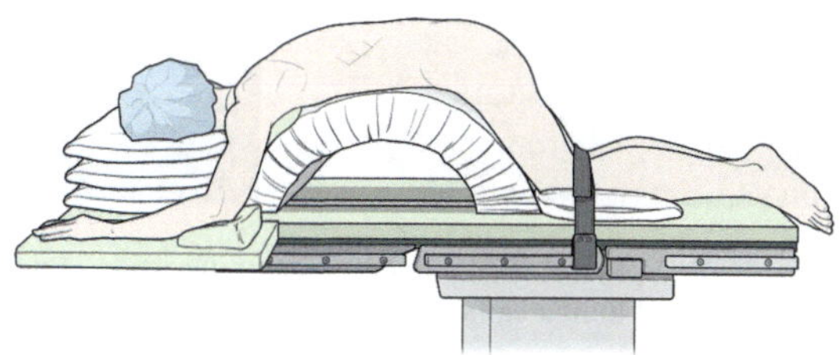

Fig. 10.4 The Wilson frame position

Step 4. Trocar Insertion

- The catheter is inserted through the trocar needle (Fig. 10.6),

Step 5. Catheter Insertion (Fig. 10.7a, b).

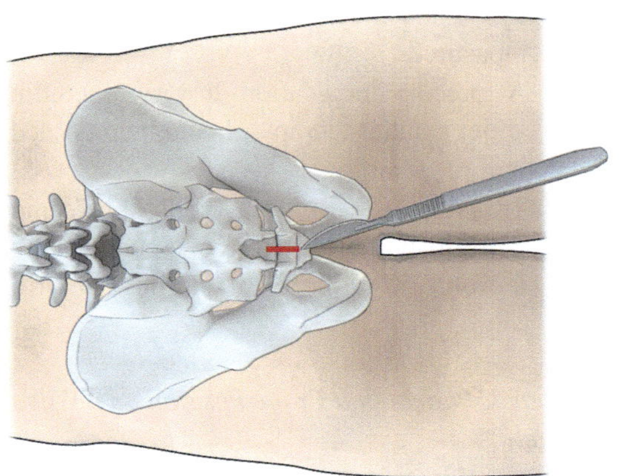

Fig. 10.5 The sacral hiatus skin incision

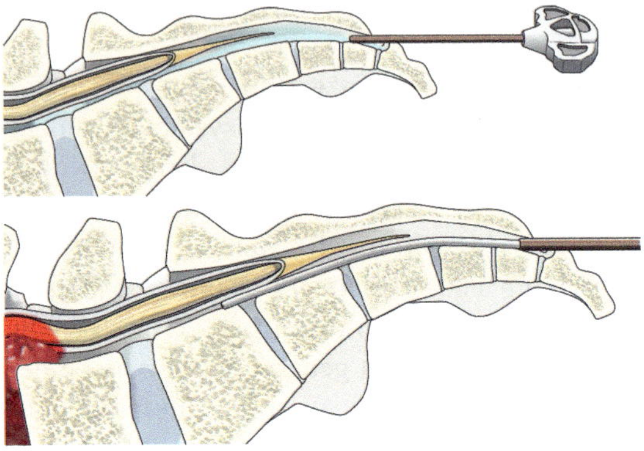

Step 6. Epidurogram (C-Arm Lateral View) for a Ventral Epidural Approach

- A bidirectional steerable catheter is inserted into the epidural space through the introduction of the trocar needle. Before inserting the

Fig. 10.6 The sacral hiatus trocar insertion

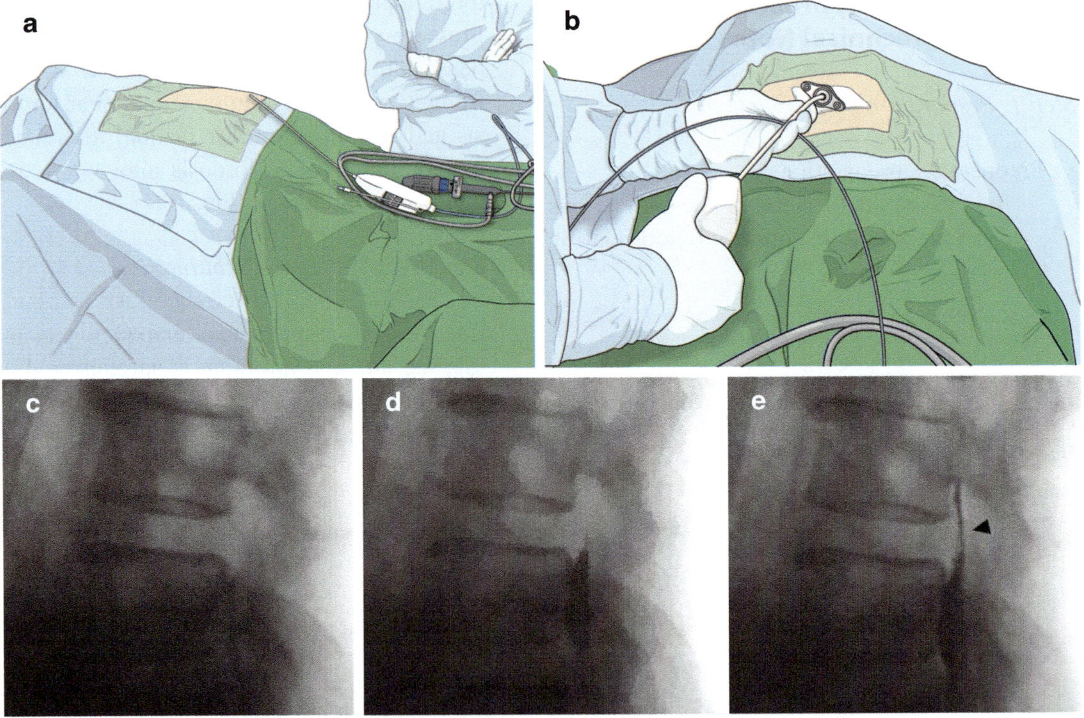

Fig. 10.7 Epidural dual lumen catheter insertion, Interoperative epidurogram. (**a**) Preparation for procedures. (**b**) Epidural dual lumen catheter insertion. (**c**, **d**, **e**) Epidurogram (Verify the position of the catheter)

catheter, 5 ml of 0.2% ropivacaine is injected through the trocar needle to reduce procedure-related pain.

- The C-arm is used to verify the position of the catheter in the ventral epidural space (Fig. 10.7c–e).
- A flexible epiduroscope is directed by the epidural catheter that was advanced to the lesion.
- The lumbar herniated disc, including inflamed tissues, engorged epidural vein, fibrous connective tissues, and epidural fat around the dura and nerve root are visualized through the epiduroscope.

Step 7. Mechanical Adhesiolysis Using Laser Ablation and Targeted Drug Delivery

- After confirming the target, the laser fiber is advanced through the bottom lumen of the catheter.
- The VersaPulse P20 laser system is used for laser ablation; the test power level is 2.5 W (0.5 J, 5 Hz), and the decompression power level is 8 W (0.8 J, 10 Hz).
- Lasering can remove perineural fibrosis, which improves local circulation and relieves pain; the laser can also penetrate and shrink the posterior longitudinal ligament and decompress the HNP.
- Laser ablation may free up fragments of the HNP; if this occurs, the laser fiber should be replaced with epiduroscopic grasping forceps to allow fragment removal.
- The position of the catheter tip should be verified using the epiduroscopic view and fluoroscopic images before performing laser ablation to prevent damage to the dura mater or spinal nerve roots.
- It is important to apply continuous irrigation to avoid a thermal injury caused by the heat generated during laser ablation.
- After laser ablation, a corticosteroid and a local anesthetic are injected into the ventral epidural space, and a mixture of hyaluronidase and hypertonic saline may also be injected for chemical adhesiolysis.

Step 8. Epidural Isotonic Fluid Irrigation.

Step 9. Normal Saline Is Continuously Infused Through the Infusion Port and Drained from the Outflow Port

- During the procedure, isotonic fluid (normal saline) is infused through the infusion port to dilate the epidural space and allow endoscopic visualization and to cool the ablation site.
- The amount and rate limitations of epidural irrigation fluids are not known;
- however, increases in epidural pressure depend on the amount of infused fluid and cause increased ICP, resulting in headaches and nuchal pain; thus, the patient should be carefully monitored.
- Epidural irrigation fluid continuously escapes through the neural foramen, and there is backflow at the drain port due to intracanal pressure; therefore, significant amounts of fluid irrigation can be injected without adverse neurological effects if the operator carefully observes the patient for changes in symptoms (Fig. 10.8).
- Patient safety recommendations include an infusion rate of 0.1–0.2 ml/s and a total saline irrigation saline volume below 200–300 ml.

Step 10. Post-Procedure Care

- We recommended an operation time of 1 h or less, as the epiduroscopic procedure can cause increased ICP.

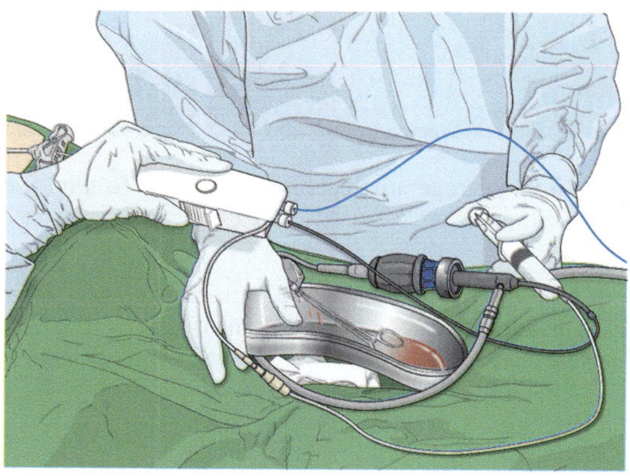

Fig. 10.8 Intraoperative procedure

- The video-guided catheter and the trocar are removed with care, and the skin is closed with one Prolene suture (Ethicon Inc., Somerville, NJ, US).
- The patient can be discharged after bed rest for the first 4 h and 24-h observation in the hospital; antibiotics and analgesics should be administered for 5 days.

10.5 Epiduroscopic Images of the Epidural Space

10.5.1 Epiduroscopic View of the Epidural Space (Fig. 10.9a–e).

10.5.2 Laser Internal Decompression of a Massive Nucleus Pulposus Herniation (C) (Fig. 10.10a–c)

10.5.3 Epiduroscopic Laser Ablation Treatment (Fig. 10.11a–g)

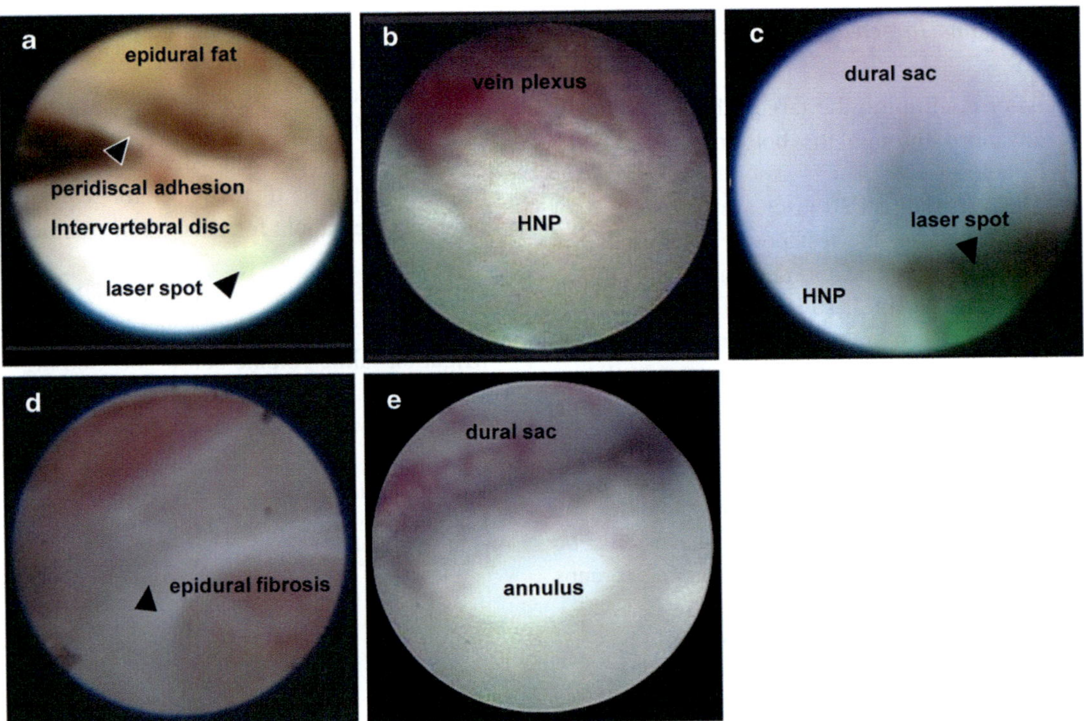

Fig. 10.9 Interoperative epiduroscopic view. (**a**) Peridiscal adhesion. (**b**) Vein plexus. (**c**) Dural sac. (**d**) Epidural fibrosis. (**e**) Annulus

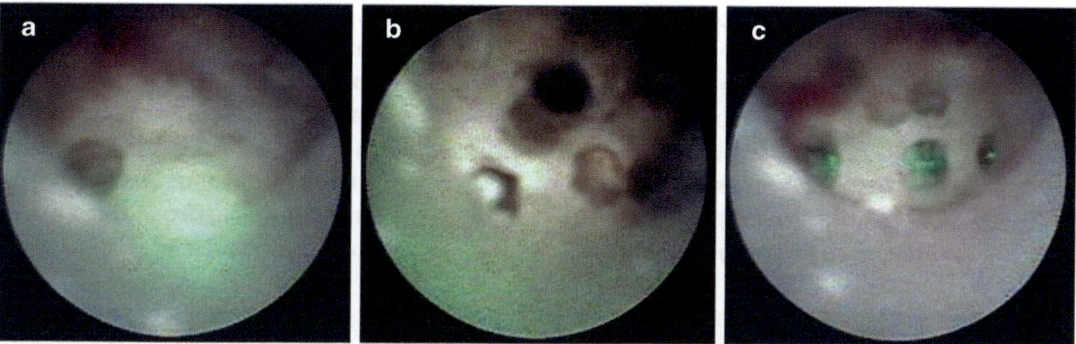

Fig. 10.10 Laser internal decompression of a massive nucleus pulposus herniation. (**a**) Place the laser tip on Herniated Nucleus Pulposus. (**b**, **c**) Laser internal decompression

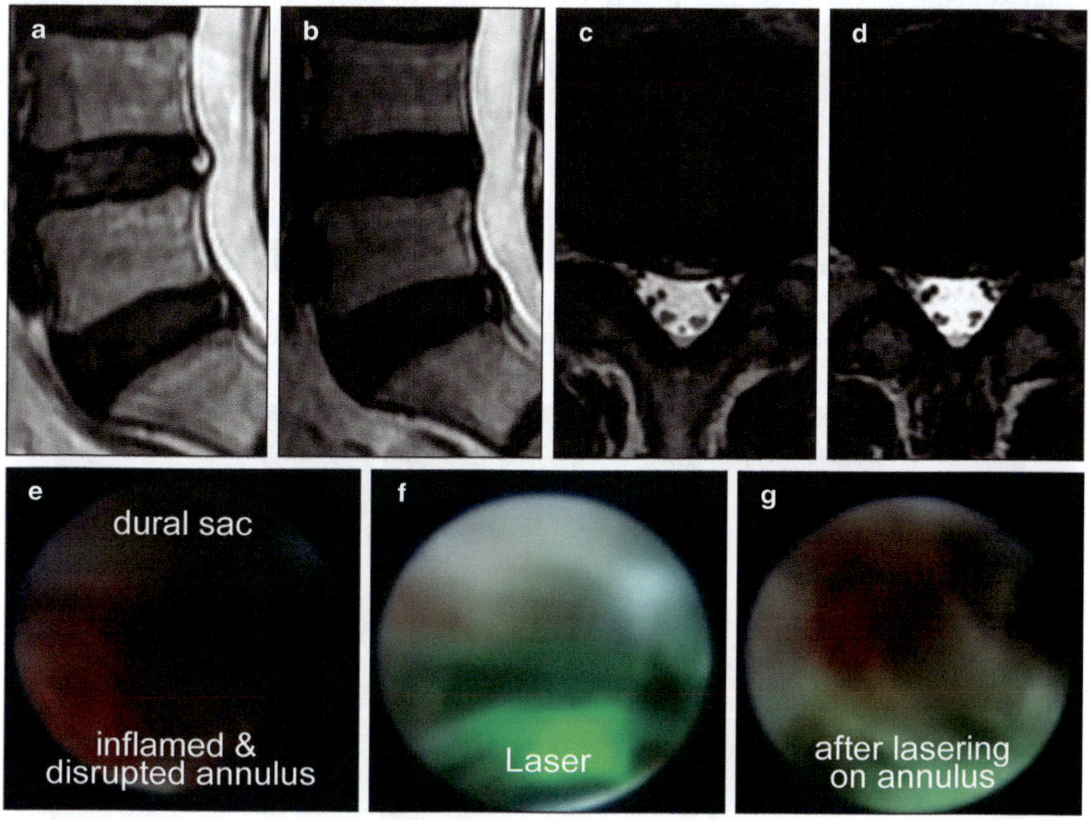

Fig. 10.11 Epiduroscopic laser treatment of a symptomatic annular tear, before (**a** and **c**) and after (**b** and **d**) treatment, an epidural, inflamed, and disrupted annulus (**e**), lasering (**f**), after lasering the annulus (**g**)

10.5.4 Supplementary Evidences

10.5.4.1 Magnetic Resonance Images Showing an Herniated Nucleus Pulposus Before and After Epiduroscopic Laser Ablation (Fig. 10.12a–b, left and right, respectively).

10.5.4.2 Epiduroscopic View During an Epiduroscopic Laser Ablation (Fig. 10.13a–f), Magnetic Resonance Images Showing a Decompressed Nucleus Pulposus Before and After Epiduroscopic Laser Ablation (Fig. 10.14a–b).

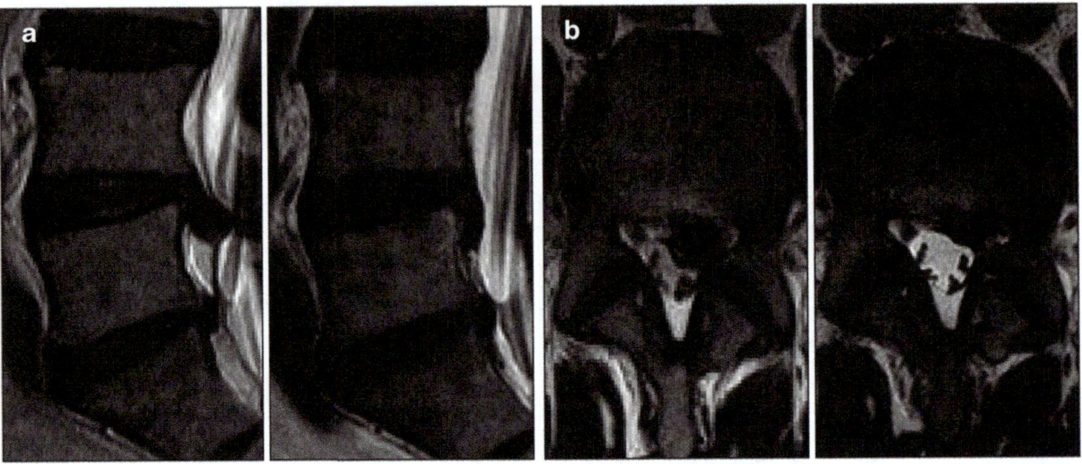

Fig. 10.12 Magnetic resonance images show an herniated nucleus pulposus before and after epiduroscopic laser ablation. (**a**) Pre-procedural Magnetic Resonance Images. (**b**) Post-procedural Magnetic Resonance Images

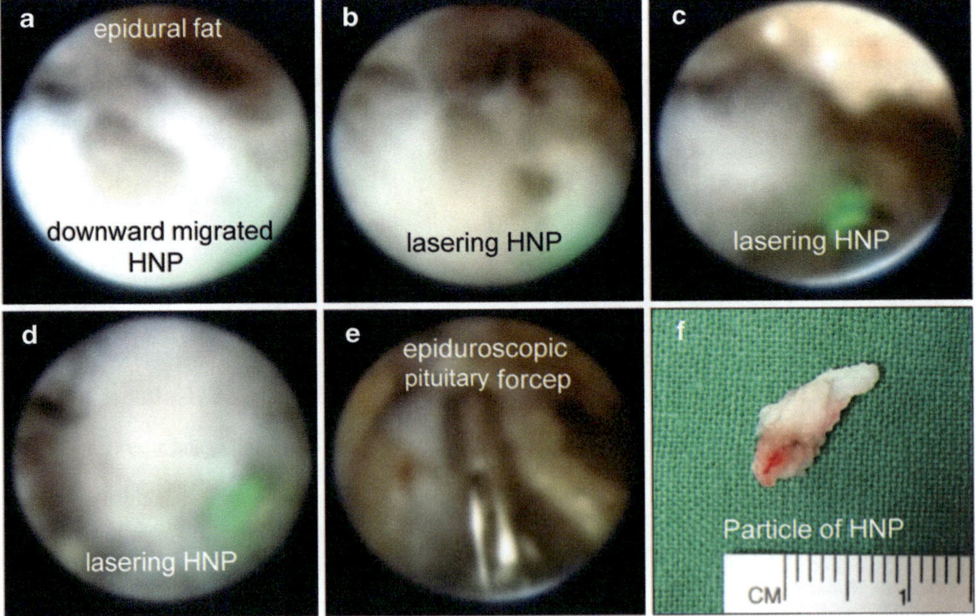

Fig. 10.13 Epiduroscopic view during a spinal procedure. (**a**) Downward migrated Herniated Nucleus Pulposus. (**b**, **c**, **d**) Lasering Herniated Nucleus Pulposus. (**e**) Removal of Herniated Nucleus Pulposus using Epiduroscopic pituitary forcep. (**f**) Removed Particle of Herniated Nucleus Pulposus

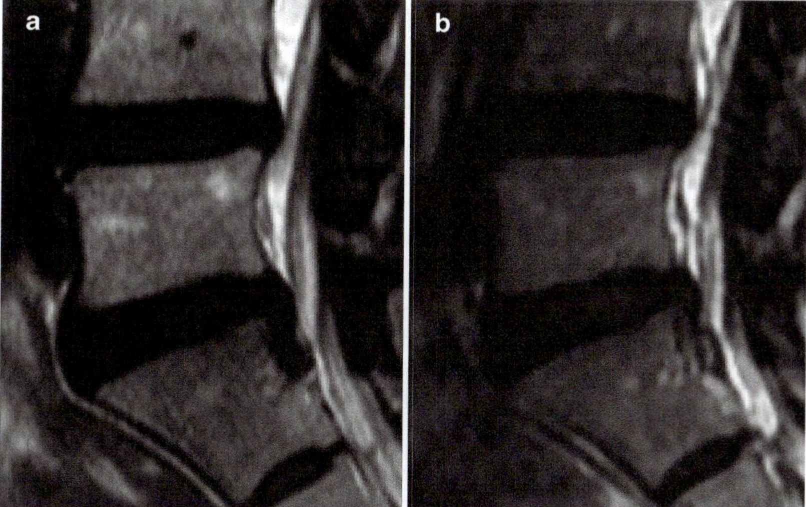

Fig. 10.14 Magnetic resonance images before and after this spinal procedure. (**a**) Pre-procedural Magnetic Resonance Images. (**b**) Post-procedural Magnetic Resonance Images

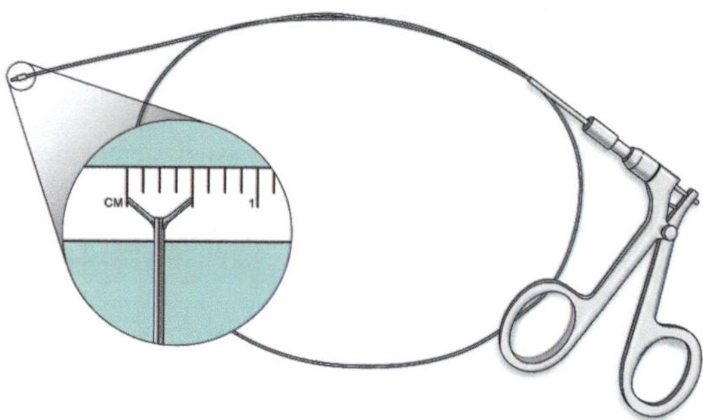

Fig. 10.15 Epiduroscopic pituitary grasping forceps

10.5.4.3 Epiduroscopic Pituitary Grasping Forceps (Fig. 10.15)

10.6 Complications

Trans-sacral discoplasty with epiduroscopy is a relatively safe, non-surgical procedure. However, like other epidural procedures, it sometimes has side effects. As more epiduroscopic procedures are being performed, the number of related complications has also increased. Operators should be familiar with the epiduroscopy-related complications listed below [13–16]:

1. Headache and nuchal pain related to increased ICP.
2. Dural tear.
3. Epidural bleeding and related hematoma.
4. Infections, including septic and aseptic discitis.
5. Epidural abscess.
6. Meningitis.
7. Temporary or permanent paresthesia and other adverse neurological outcomes.
8. Pneumocephalus.
9. Incomplete or failed procedure.
10. Recurrent disc herniation.
11. Visual disturbances secondary to rapid epidural saline infusion.

10.7 Conclusion

Epiduroscopy is widely used, and epiduroscopic techniques have been developed for the treatment of pain originating from spinal disorders. Trans-sacral epiduroscopy is a very useful treatment for patients with LBP and radicular leg pain. The procedure has a low complication rate, an immediate therapeutic effect, and a short rehabilitation period that allows a swift return to normal daily activities.

In the future, epiduroscopes will be thinner, the steering catheter will be more versatile, and the epiduroscopic image quality will be further improved. Therefore, trans-sacral epiduroscopic procedures will continue to play an important role as effective, non-surgical treatment for spinal pain.

References

1. Fyneface-Ogan S. Anatomy and clinical importance of the epidural space. In. Epidural analgesia-current views and approaches. IntechOpen. 2012.
2. Hogan QH. Epidural anatomy: new observations. Can J Anaesth. 1998;45(5 Pt 2):R40–8.
3. Alò K, Abramova M, Redko V, Williams J, McKee M, Noto D. Technical update in spinal mapping, epidural disc and neural decompression, and neurostimulation: an interventional continuum for axial and radicular pain. In: Minimally invasive surgery for pain, vol. II. Southern Academic Press; 2013.
4. Blomberg RG, Olsson SS. The lumbar epidural space in patients examined with epiduroscopy. Anesth Analg. 1989;68:157–60.
5. Oh CH, Ji GY, Cho PG, Choi WS, Shin DA, Kim KN, et al. The catheter tip position and effects of percutaneous epidural neuroplasty in patients with lumbar disc disease during 6-months of follow-up. Pain Physician. 2014;17:E599–608.
6. Burman MS. Myeloscopy or the direct visualization of the spinal canal and its contents. J Bone Joint Surg. 1931;13:695–6.
7. Pool JL. Direct visualization of dorsal nerve roots of the cauda equina by means of a myeloscope. Arch Neur Psych. 1938;39:1308–12.
8. Leu H. Percutaneous techniques: decompression and intradiscal laser in discoscopy, external pedicular fixation, percutaneous interbody fusion, peridural endoscopy with discoscopy. 12th course of percutaneous endoscopic spinal surgery, Zürich; 1993.
9. Ooi Y, Morisaki N. Intrathecal lumbar endoscope. Clin Ortop Surg (Japan). 1969;4:295–7.
10. Saberski LR, Kitahata LM. Direct visualization of the lumbosacral epidural space through the sacral hiatus. Anesth Analg. 1995;80:839–40.
11. Takeshima N, Miyakawa H, Okuda K, Hattori S, Hagiwara S, Takatani J, et al. Evaluation of the therapeutic results of epiduroscopic adhesiolysis for failed back surgery syndrome. Br J Anaesth. 2009;102:400–7.
12. Moon BJ, Lee HY, Kim KN, Yi S, Ha Y, Yoon DH, et al. Experimental evaluation of percutaneous lumbar laser disc decompression using a 1414 nm Nd: YAG laser. Pain Physician. 2015;18:E1091–9.
13. Richter EO, Abramova MV, Cantu F, DeAndres J, Lierz P, PierLuigi M, et al. Anterior epiduroscopic neural decompression: eight-center experience in 154 patients. Eur J Pain Suppl. 2012;5:401–7.
14. Avellanal M, Diaz-Reganon G, Orts A, Gonzalez-Montero L, Ares JDA. Epiduroscopy: complications and troubleshooting. Tech Reg Anesth Pain Manag. 2014;18:35–9.
15. Epstein JM, Adler R. Laser-assisted percutaneous endoscopic neurolysis. Pain Physician. 2000;3:43–5.
16. Heavner JE, Bosscher HA. Complications of lumbosacral epiduroscopy. Pain Clin. 2007;19:178–84.

11 Manual Percutaneous Foraminoplasty

Kyung-Woo Park and Sang-Heon Lee

11.1 Introduction

Although studies describe the lumbar spine transforaminal ligaments (TFLs), their clinical implications are unclear as they do not typically affect many surgical conditions [1, 2] (Figs. 11.1 and 11.2).

However, stenosis caused by disc space narrowing decreases the size of the intervertebral foramen, thus increasing the relative size of the TFLs. In their anatomical studies, Min et al. observed that TFLs frequently trapped exiting nerves [3], which could explain persistent radicular pain occurring postsurgical decompression. The increasing use of the posterolateral approach to lateral disc herniations emphasizes the anatomical importance of the TFLs.

TFLs can be assigned to four categories based on their anatomic locations, namely, the entrance zone, mid-zone, exit zone, and post-canal zone ligaments. The ligaments of the entrance zone include the posterior longitudinal ligament, Hofmann's ligament, and the peridural membrane; the ligaments of the mid-zone include fascial condensations that attach the nerve root sleeve to the vertebral arch pedicles and ligamentum flavum; the ligaments of the exit zone (around the intervertebral foramen) include the internal, transforaminal, and external ligaments (Fig. 11.3); and the post-canal zone contains the lumbar cribriform fascia [4].

In contrast, Amonoo-Kuofi et al. described three TFL categories, namely, the internal, intraforaminal, and external ligaments. The internal ligament group includes the oblique inferior TFL; the intraforaminal ligament group includes the deep anterior intraforaminal ligament, the oblique superior TFL, and the horizontal mid-TFL; and the external ligament group includes the superior, middle, and inferior corporotransverse ligaments. However, a different classification is applied to the L5–S1 intervertebral foramina [3] (Figs. 11.4 and 11.5). The L5–S1 intervertebral foramen contains four ligamentous structures: the lumbosacral ligament, the lumbosacral hood, the corporotransverse ligament, and the mamillo-transverso-accessory ligament.

Foraminal stenosis may entrap the L1–L4 dorsal root ganglions (DRG) by the superior and inferior corporotransverse ligaments and the L5 DRG by the corporotransverse ligament. In addi-

K.-W. Park (✉)
Kwanghye Spine Hospital, Seoul, Republic of Korea

S.-H. Lee
Department of Spine and Pain Center, Korea University Anam Hospital, Seoul, Republic of Korea

S.-H. Lee (ed.), *Minimally Invasive Spine Interventions*,
https://doi.org/10.1007/978-981-16-9547-6_11

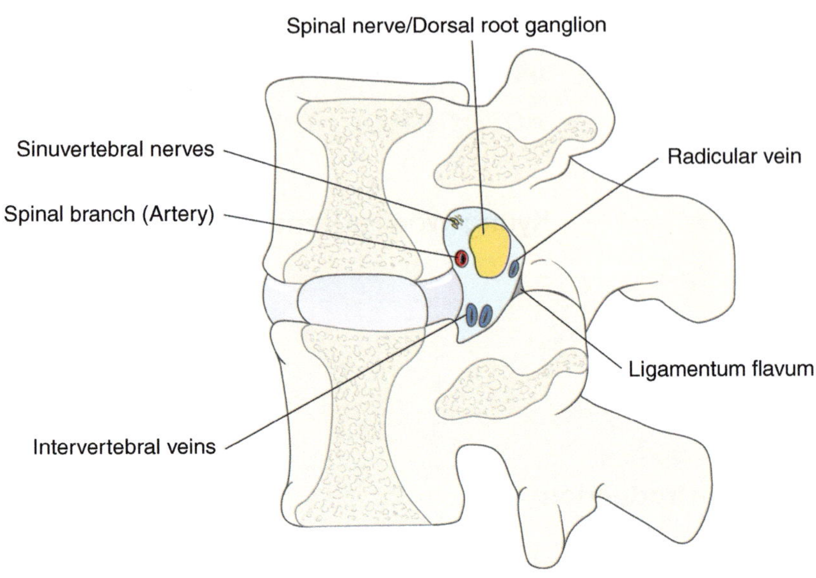

Fig. 11.1 An illustration of the clinical anatomy of the intervertebral foramen. The components include the spinal nerve (dorsal root ganglion), sinuvertebral nerves, radicular and intervertebral veins, spinal artery, and ligaments

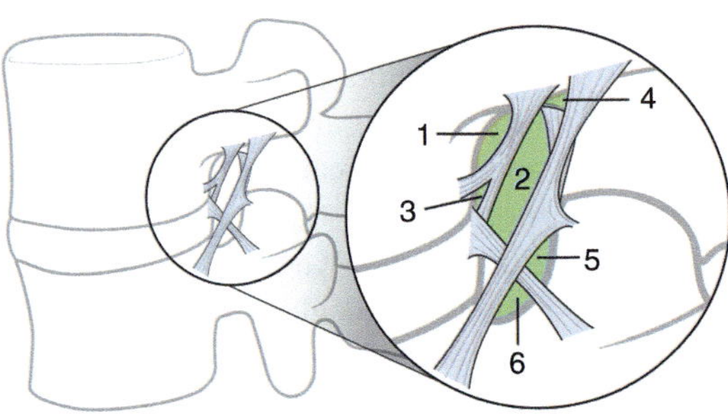

Fig. 11.2 A schematic diagram showing the external aspect of the intervertebral foramen, including the spinal artery (1), ventral ramus of the spinal nerve (2), recurrent meningeal nerve (3), medial (4) and lateral (5) divisions of the dorsal primary ramus, and veins (6)

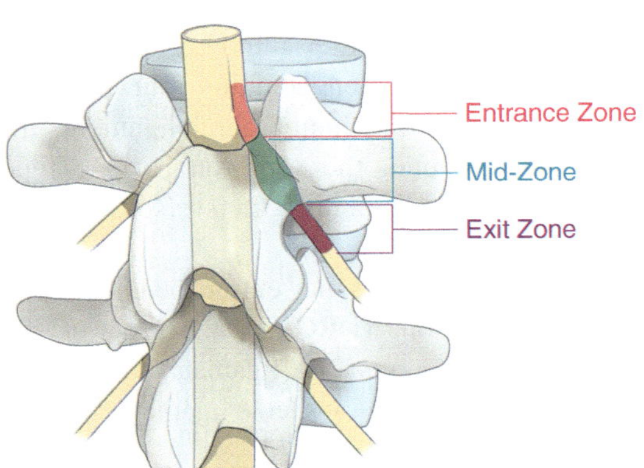

Fig. 11.3 An illustration of the clinical anatomy of the transforaminal ligaments

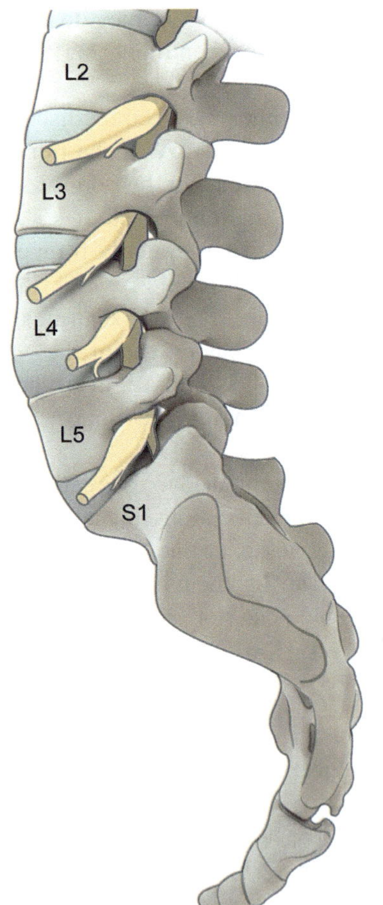

Fig. 11.4 An illustration showing the anatomy of the ligaments that cross the intervertebral foramen

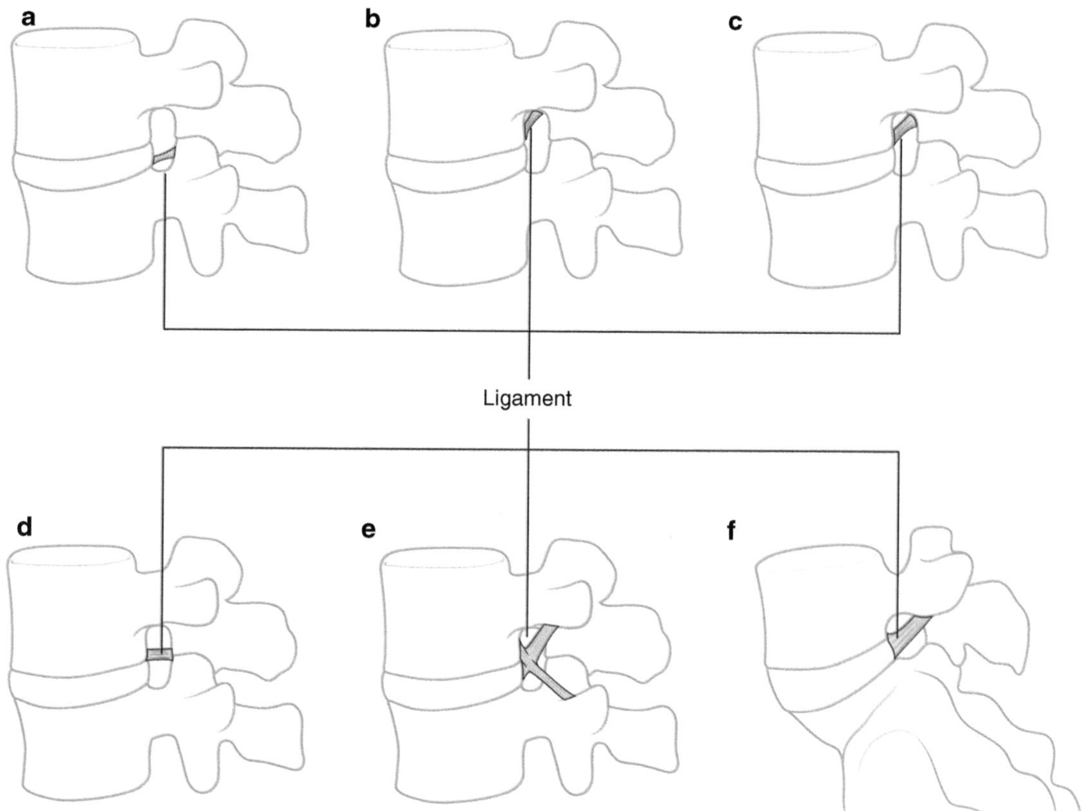

Fig. 11.5 Illustrations showing the clinical anatomy of the ligaments that cross the intervertebral foramen. These ligaments show anatomical variability: oblique inferior transforaminal ligament (**a**), anterior intraforaminal ligament (**b**), oblique superior transforaminal ligament (**c**), mid-transforaminal ligament (**d**), superior and inferior corporotransverse ligaments (**e**), and corporotransverse ligament (**f**)

tion, foraminal ligament ossification and trunk and conjoint nerve roots increase the likelihood of DRG entrapment. The resulting recurrent inflammation creates adhesive fibrosis, both of which may cause low back, buttock, and leg pain.

11.2 Background

Neurolysis using hypertonic saline and hyaluronidase, as well as purported adhesion lysis by percutaneous-directed catheters, do not decompress DRG entrapped by TFLs. Thus, surgical decompression is required.

In this context, Kyung-Woo Park (Seoul, South Korea) invented a set of instruments to perform percutaneous foraminoplasty with foraminal ligament resection and adhesion decompression [5]. Percutaneous foraminoplasty expands the size of intervertebral foramina that have been narrowed or blocked by adhesive fibrosis resulting from recurrent inflammatory reactions. The procedure involves the resection of minute ligaments entangled in the intervertebral foramen, delivery of pain medications to the periphery of pain-generating nerve branches, and removal of inflammatory materials from the spinal canal through the intervertebral foramen.

11.3 Effectiveness of Percutaneous Foraminoplasty with Ligament Resection

11.3.1 Introduction

Lumbar foraminal spinal stenosis (LFSS) is defined as the narrowing of the nerve root exit caused by a decrease in the height of an intervertebral disk, osteoarthritic changes in the facet joints, cephalad subluxation of the superior articular process (SAP) of the inferior vertebra, buckling of the ligamentum flavum, or protrusion of the AF in the lumbar spinal canal [6–8]. Despite a paucity of studies examining the mechanical compression of nerve roots in LFSS, it has been assumed that LFSS results in damage to microvascular structures and continuous compression of nerve roots, subsequently causing ischemia, edema, demyelination, and C-fiber hyperactivation [9, 10].

Although various minimally invasive procedures have been considered for managing radicular pain caused by LFSS in patients refractory to oral medication and physical therapy, their ability to provide effective pain relief in this population is questionable. Lumbar transforaminal epidural steroid injection (TFESI) is the most widely used treatment; however, it shows less effectiveness in lumbar spinal stenosis compared to that in disc herniation and may not improve the average impairment of function [11, 12]. Percutaneous epidural adhesiolysis is another option for managing patients with lumbar spinal stenosis [13–15]. However, previous studies suggest a negative outcome for patients with LFSS, spondylolisthesis, and previous lumbar surgery [14]. Although spinal cord stimulation may guarantee a positive outcome after a successful trial in lumbar spinal stenosis, there has been a paucity of information about the outcome in patients with LFSS, and the high initial cost is still burdensome [16, 17]. As a last resort, surgical decompression such as laminotomy, laminectomy, medial facetectomy, or endoscopic foraminotomy can be considered in patients refractory to previous conservative treatments; however, a recent review failed to prove the short- or long-term superiority of these lumbar spinal surgeries compared to conservative care at follow-up [18–22].

One hypothesis of the physiopathology of LFSS is that numerous lumbar foraminal ligaments cause LBP and radiculopathy [3, 23–25]. The lumbar foraminal ligaments include the superior and inferior TFLs and superior and inferior corporotransverse (or corporopedicular) ligaments [9, 23]. These structures fix the lumbosacral spinal nerves to the intervertebral foramen and protect the nerve and blood vessels from damage. However, abnormal adhesions and excess TFLs may result in pain through the compression of the nerve root [25].

A specially designed instrument for percutaneous foraminoplasty was invented to allow a minimally invasive procedure. This procedure aims to achieve effective decompression of structures affected by LFSS by resecting foraminal ligaments and facilitating the spread of medication around the target nerve. The purpose of this study was to evaluate the effectiveness of percutaneous foraminoplasty in patients with intractable radiculopathy from LFSS.

11.3.2 Methods

This prospective, single-armed, observational pilot study was approved by the institutional review board at the participating hospital (Seoul National University Hospital IRB No. 1311-067-534) and was conducted in accordance with the ethical principles of the Declaration of Helsinki. This study was registered in Clinical Trials (NCT02597244) before initiating the study-related procedures. Patient enrollment took place from September 2014 to January 2016. Written informed consent was obtained from all patients before their participation in the study.

11.3.3 Patients

The inclusion criteria were (1) patients 45–85 years of age with chronic lumbar radicular pain at the L4 or L5 dermatome; (2) concordant imaging evidence of LFSS (grades 1–3; mild, moderate, and severe LFSS, respectively) as demonstrated on preoperative magnetic resonance imaging (MRI) scans [26]; (3) failed pain relief or short-term pain relief for 1 month or less from a previous TFESI; (4) patients with numerical rating scale (NRS) pain scores (0: no pain, 10: worst pain possible) of >4 out of 10 despite appropriate conservative treatment including physiotherapy, exercise therapy, or oral medications for at least 6 months; and (5) patients with single-side radiculopathy.

The exclusion criteria were (1) patients with complaints of dominant back pain rather than leg pain; (2) lack of correlation between radicular pain and MRI findings; (3) history of prior lumbar spine surgery or any previous percutaneous foraminoplasty procedure; (4) iliac crest located higher than the L5 transverse process, which would disturb the lateral approach to the L5 foramen during the percutaneous foraminoplasty procedure; (5) progressive neurological deficits, motor weakness, or cauda equina syndrome; (6) allergies to steroids or contrast dyes; (7) clinical signs of spinal cord compression, bleeding disorders, infection, instability, malignancy or other traumatic injuries, poorly controlled coexisting psychiatric conditions, or underlying systemic diseases; and (8) pregnancy.

The administration of oral or transdermal analgesics such as opioids, tramadol, or nonsteroidal anti-inflammatory drugs (NSAIDs) was allowed to continue during the study. In addition, the dosages of these medications as rescue or regular (around-the-clock) analgesics were modified appropriately according to the pain intensity. Adjuvants such as anticonvulsants and antidepressants that were used to manage radicular pain were also continued. In the first month post-percutaneous foraminoplasty, any additional medication or therapy, including physical therapy, trigger point injections, and EIs, was not allowed. After the first visit, the patients were allowed to undergo physical therapy or interventional procedures other than ESIs, such as TFESI, and take additional medication including NSAIDs, antidepressants, anticonvulsants, and opioids.

11.3.4 Clinical Evaluation

This open-labeled observational study included a baseline visit before percutaneous foraminoplasty (Visit 0) and follow-ups at 1, 2, and 3 months (Visits 1, 2, and 3, respectively). The NRS pain score at each visit was calculated as the average of the NRS pain scores for radicular leg pain during the previous week [27]. After the percutaneous foraminoplasty procedure, the enrolled patients were encouraged to record a daily diary during the follow-up period. The Korean versions of the nine-item Oswestry Disability Index (ODI [range, 0–100, where 0 means no disability]) and the Roland-Morris Disability Questionnaire (RMDQ [range, 0–24, where 0 means no disability]) were also used to evaluate the physical function at each visit [28, 29]. One research nurse who was independent of the study conducted all assessments.

The primary endpoint of the study was the percentage of successful responders at Visit 3. This indicator was determined according to previous studies, with some modifications such as a reduction of 40% or more compared to the baseline NRS pain score and no increase from baseline ODI and RMDQ scores at Visit 3 [30–33]. Furthermore, increased dosage of analgesics, the prescription of new analgesics, and the administration of an additional ESI during the follow-up period were all considered treatment failure.

Changes in the 11-point NRS score for radicular pain, ODI score, and RMDQ score at the 3-month follow-up (Visit 3) compared to baseline (Visit 0) were analyzed for responding and nonresponding patients. In addition, overall changes in NRS pain score, ODI, and RMDQ score over time were compared between responding and nonresponding patients. The patients were prescribed oral analgesics at each visit and encouraged to record their consumption of medication in a daily diary throughout the study period. At Visit 3, the consumption of oral medication, including NSAIDs, opioids, antidepressants, and anticonvulsants, was compared to baseline consumption in each patient. Finally, patient satisfaction with the extraforaminotomy (EF) procedure was assessed using a five-point

Likert satisfaction scale (1, extremely dissatisfied; 2, somewhat dissatisfied; 3, neutral; 4, somewhat satisfied; and 5, extremely satisfied) at Visit 3.

The patients were asked to report any adverse events of the transforaminal extraforaminotomy (TFEF) during the study period. The reported adverse events were noted and evaluated at each visit.

11.3.5 Statistical Analysis

Efficacy analyses were performed on the per-protocol population for the primary and secondary endpoints, while safety analysis was performed on the intent-to-treat population.

The differences between responding and non-responding patients were tested using the Mann-Whitney and Fisher's exact tests for nonparametric and parametric data, respectively. Wilcoxon signed-rank tests were used to assess the statistical significance of differences between the NRS, ODI, and RMDQ scores at Visit 3 and at the baseline. Subsequently, a general linear mixed-model analysis for longitudinal data was also performed.

Data were analyzed with IBM SPSS Statistics for Windows, version 22.0 (IBM Corp, Armonk, NY, US). The outcomes are shown as means (interquartile range [IQR] or standard deviation) or frequencies (%) as appropriate. *P*-values <0.05 were considered statistically significant.

11.3.6 Results

We recruited 35 patients who had been diagnosed with LFSS between September 2014 and September 2015. Among them, 26 patients were enrolled and underwent percutaneous foraminoplasty. However, six patients dropped out during the 3-month follow-up. Hence, 20 patients completed the study protocol, and follow-up data were collected at 1, 2, and 3 months [34] (Fig. 11.6).

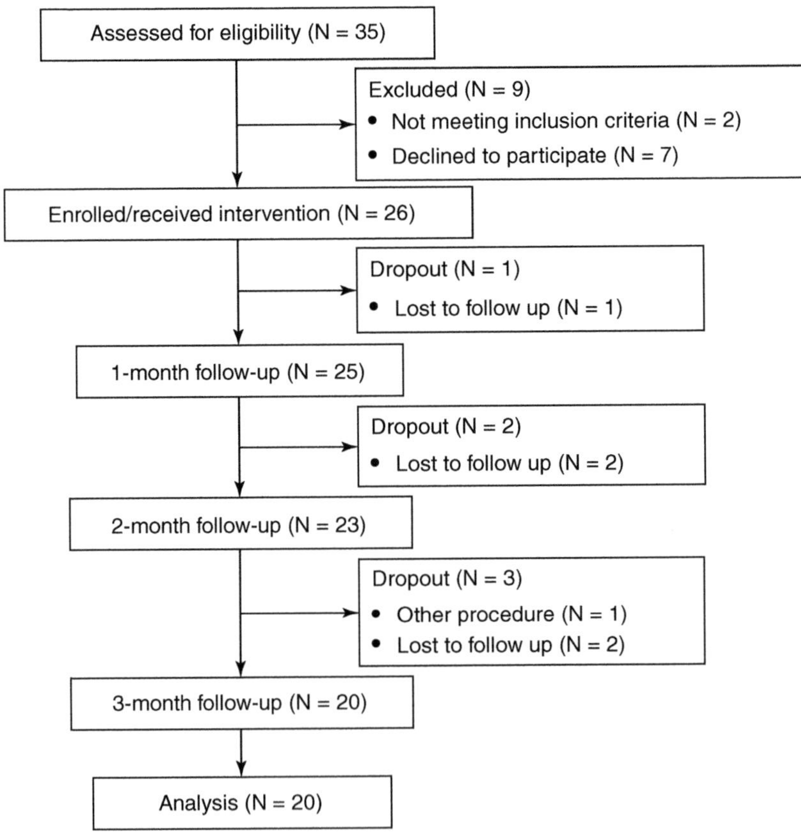

Fig. 11.6 Flowchart of study patients

The baseline patient demographic characteristics, including a comparison between responders and nonresponders, are shown in Table 11.1. Within the cohort, most ($N = 14$, 70%) underwent percutaneous foraminoplasty at the L4–L5 transforaminal space [34]. The baseline NRS pain score for the lower extremities was 6.60 (IQR, 5.0–8.0), indicating moderate to severe pain. The mean ODI (%) and RMDQ scores were 65.55 (IQR, 53.3–72.8) and 12.60 (IQR, 6.0–15.0), respectively, suggesting that pain affected all aspects of the patients' lives [33, 35]. No statistically significant differences between responders and nonresponders were observed in the demographic and clinical variables. The only exception was the number of patients receiving opioid medication. Three patients in the nonresponder group were prescribed a weak opioid, tramadol, and acetaminophen mixture, a significant difference compared to the responder group ($N = 0$, $P = 0.049$). In the overall cohort, none of the patients had taken strong opioid medication.

Twelve patients (60%) reported a successful response to the percutaneous foraminoplasty procedure, with at least a 40% pain reduction and no increase from baseline ODI and RMDQ score at Visit 3. Table 11.2 shows the overall changes in NRS pain scores for the legs, ODI (%), and RMDQ score at the 3-month follow-up, including a comparison between responders and nonresponders. The mean pain reduction (%) at 3 months was 36.3% overall. All scores at 3 months were significantly lower than those at baseline in the responding and nonresponding patients; nonetheless, this difference was also significant between the groups.

Figure 11.7 shows that the NRS pain scores, ODI (%), and RMDQ scores decreased significantly over time compared to the baseline values (all $P < 0.001$ in the general linear mixed model analysis for repeated measures) [34]. Regarding patient satisfaction, 65% of patients were "extremely satisfied" or "somewhat satisfied" with the percutaneous foraminoplasty procedure

Table 11.1 Baseline patient characteristics and demographics

Parameters	Value ($N = 20$)	Responders ($N = 12$)	Nonresponders ($N = 8$)	P
Age (y)	67.6 (60.3–73.8)	69.8 (65.3–74.0)	64.3 (58.5–66.8)	0.115
Sex (male/female)	7 (35.0)/13 (65.0)	5/7	2/6	0.642
Height (cm)	160.7 (153.4–167.6)	161.5 (153.9–169.0)	159.5 (149.1–167.1)	0.624
Weight (kg)	64.6 (58.2–74.3)	66.3 (55.9–75.8)	62.2 (58.2–69.5)	0.343
Hypertension	13 (65.0)	9 (75.0)	4 (50.0)	0.356
Total duration of pain (months)	12.0 (8.0–14.0)	11.2 (8.0–14.0)	13.1 (8.3–18.0)	0.305
Level, L4–5/L5–S1 vertebrae	14 (70.0)/6 (30.0)	7/5	7/1	0.325
Side (left/right)	10 (50.0)/10 (50.0)	6/6	4/4	0.370
LFSS grade I/II/III	8 (40.0)/9 (45)/3 (15.0)	5/6/1	3/3/2	0.584
Previous epidural injection	3.7 (2.3–5.0)	3.1 (1.3–5.0)	4.5 (3.3–5.0)	0.157
NRS leg pain score (0–10)	6.6 (5.0–8.0)	7.1 (5.0–8.8)	5.9 (5.0–6.8)	0.157
ODI (%)	65.6 (53.3–72.8)	64.8 (53.3–71.1)	66.7 (52.8–84.4)	0.427
RMDQ score (0–24)	12.6 (6.0–15.0)	12.1 (6.0–14.8)	13.2 (6.5–18.0)	0.970
Analgesic use				
Non-NSAIDs[a]	8 (40.0)	4 (33.3)	4 (50.0)	0.648
NSAIDs	10 (50.0)	5 (41.7)	5 (62.5)	0.650
Opioids	3 (15.0)	0 (0.0)	3 (37.5)	0.049

Data are expressed as numbers (%) or medians (interquartile range)
L lumbar, *LFSS* lumbar foraminal spinal stenosis, *NRS* numerical rating scale, *NSAID* nonsteroidal anti-inflammatory drug, *ODI* Oswestry Disability Index, *RMDQ* Roland-Morris Disability Questionnaire, *S* sacral
[a] Non-NSAIDs include antidepressants and anticonvulsants

Table 11.2 Clinical outcomes of responder analysis at the 3-month follow-up

Variables	Total (N = 20)	Responders (N = 12)	Nonresponders (N = 8)	P
NRS pain score at 3 m	−2.6 (−4.0–−1.0)	−4.1 (−4.8–−3.0)	−0.4 (−1.0–0.0)	<0.001
Changes in NRS from baseline at 3 months (%)	−36.3 (−15.7–−54.2)	−57.0 (−45.8–−71.3)	−5.4 (−20.0–0.0)	<0.001
ODI (%) at 3 months	−13.3 (−21.7–−5.0)	−19.9 (−25.6–−11.1)	−3.6 (−10.0–3.3)	0.002
RMDQ score at 3 months, 0–24	−6.2 (−8.0–−3.3)	−8.4 (−12.3–−11.1)	−2.9 (−6.8–0.8)	0.020
Analgesic use				
Non-NSAIDs[a]	−3 (5, 20%)	−2 (2, 16.7%)	−1 (3, 37.5%)	0.347
NSAIDs	−1 (9, 45%)	−2 (3, 25.0%)	+ 1 (6, 75.0%)	0.065
Opioids	−1 (2, 10%)	0 (0, 0.0%)	−1 (2, 25.0%)	0.147
Satisfaction (1 or 2 on the five-point Likert scale)[b]	13 (65)	10 (83.3)	3 (37.5)	0.062

Data are expressed as numbers (%) or medians (interquartile range)

NRS numerical rating scale, *NSAID* nonsteroidal anti-inflammatory drug, *ODI* Oswestry Disability Index, *RMDQ* Roland-Morris Disability Questionnaire

[a]Non-NSAIDs include antidepressants and anticonvulsants

[b]Patient satisfaction with the extraforaminotomy procedure was assessed using the five-point Likert satisfaction scale (1, extremely dissatisfied; 2, somewhat dissatisfied; 3, neutral; 4, somewhat satisfied; 5, extremely satisfied) at Visit 3

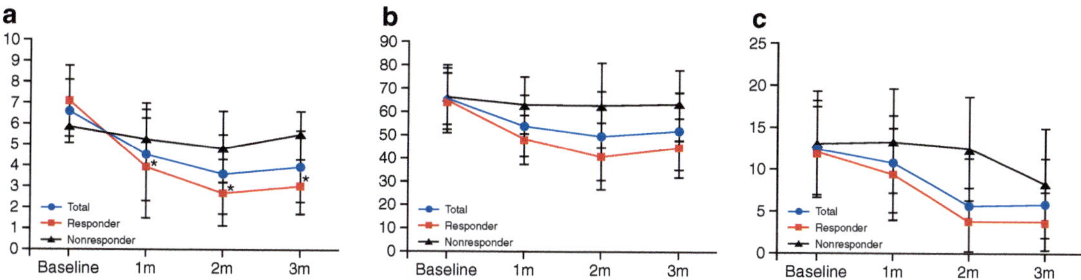

Fig. 11.7 Changes in numerical rating scale leg pain scores, including the Oswestry Disability Index (%) (**a**) and Roland-Morris Disability Questionnaire score (**b**). *$P < 0.05$ compared to baseline (**c**)

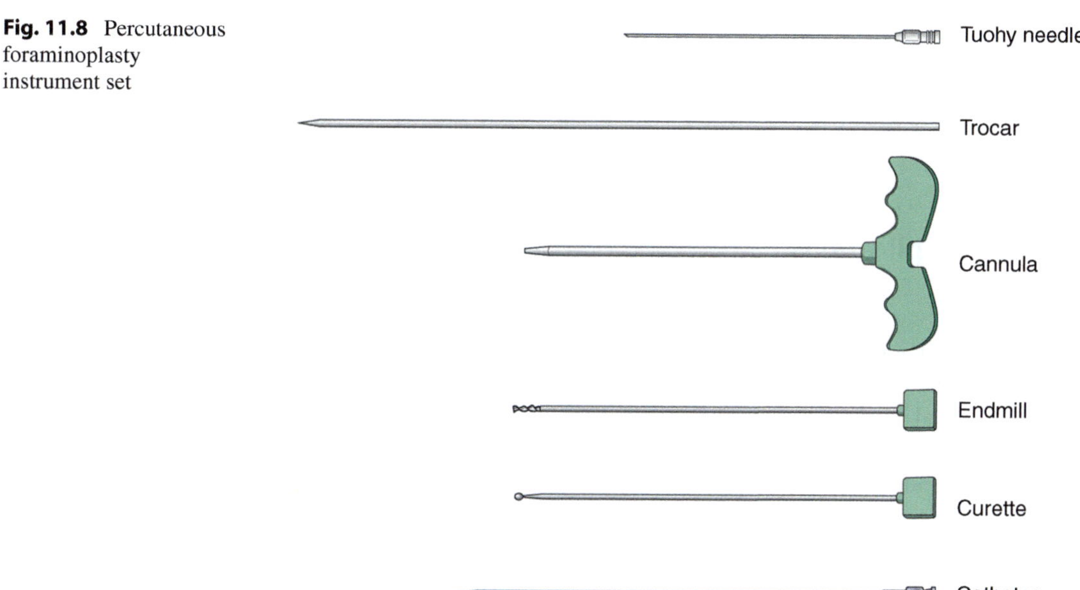

Fig. 11.8 Percutaneous foraminoplasty instrument set

(Table 11.2), while four patients were "neutral," and two patients were "somewhat dissatisfied." None of the patients were "extremely dissatisfied" with the procedure. Although the overall use of analgesics was reduced at 3 months, we observed no statistically significant difference between responding and nonresponding patients [34].

All adverse events that occurred during the study period were minor and temporary. Most ($N = 13$, 65%) of the patients reported temporary pain during the procedure, which was tolerable and did not require additional medication or discontinuation of the procedure. Nine patients complained of procedure-related pain for 2 to 3 days in the postprocedural period, which spontaneously resolved without any neurological sequelae. Three patients reported transient paresthesia in the lower extremities that resolved within 1 week. No other adverse events, such as dural puncture, hematoma formation, persistent motor or sensory impairment, severe pain, paresthesia, or infection, were reported (Fig. 11.8).

11.3.7 Discussion

The results of this prospective pilot study showed that the percutaneous foraminoplasty procedure was successful in 60% ($N = 12$) of appropriately selected patients with radicular pain secondary to LFSS. Additionally, the patients who responded well also showed functional improvement, as assessed by the ODI (%) and RMDQ score, at the 3-month follow-up. No serious complications were reported in the study. Presumably, the percutaneous foraminoplasty procedure alleviates LFSS symptoms by mechanically eliminating adhesions of the ligamentous structures that may compress exiting nerve roots, reducing venous stasis, decreasing perineural edema, and eventually promoting the spread of injectate [23, 25]. Percutaneous foraminoplasty targets adhesiolysis, particularly at the posterior and inferior quadrants of the neural foramen, using the rounded rim of a cannula, the blunt edge portion of the end mill, and a cup-shaped curette. These objects were designed to minimize damage to the surrounding tissue, such as the dura, DRG, and blood vessels.

11.4 Complications

Although a few patients experienced temporary dysesthesia after the procedure, perhaps due to irritation of the exiting nerve root, this was completely relieved within 2 to 3 days. The mechanical elimination of adhesions requires repetitive advancement and withdrawal of the instrument, which may have caused procedure-related pain and a risk of bleeding during the percutaneous foraminoplasty procedure.

11.5 Conclusions

Percutaneous foraminoplasty with ligament resection performed using a specially designed instrument set is a safe treatment option that effectively reduced the intensity of refractory LBP. Further, this minimally invasive procedure may facilitate the functional recovery of the intervertebral foramen because the novel instrument set is designed to affect only extremely small TFLs and minimize damage to the surrounding tissues such as the dura (DRG), blood vessels, and bones (facet joint and lamina). I hope that this procedure will become the cornerstone of the minimally invasive spinal intervention that I call the "out-in approach for IVF."

References

1. Kim DH, Choi G. Endoscopic spine procedures. New York: Thieme; 2011.
2. Amonoo-Kuofi HS, el-Badawi MG, Fatani JA. Ligaments associated with lumbar intervertebral foramina. 1. L1 to L4. J Anat. 1988;156:177–83.
3. Min JH, Kang SH, Lee JB, Cho TH, Suh JG. Anatomic analysis of the transforaminal ligament in the lumbar intervertebral foramen. Neurosurgery. 2005;57:37–41. discussion 37–41
4. Giles L. Ligaments traversing the intervertebral canals of the human lower lumbosacral spine. Neuro Orthop. 1992;13:25–38.
5. Park KW. Percutaneous extraforaminotomy with foraminal ligament resection and instrument tool used for the same. In: Google Patents; 2017. https://patents.google.com/patent/US9649129B2/en. Accessed.
6. Hasegawa T, An HS, Haughton VM, Nowicki BH. Lumbar foraminal stenosis: critical heights of the intervertebral discs and foramina. A cryomicrotome study in cadavera. J Bone Joint Surg Am. 1995;77:32–8.
7. Splendiani A, Ferrari F, Barile A, Masciocchi C, Gallucci M. Occult neural foraminal stenosis caused by association between disc degeneration and facet joint osteoarthritis: demonstration with dedicated upright MRI system. Radiol Med. 2014;119:164–74.
8. Jenis LG, An HS. Spine update. Lumbar foraminal stenosis. Spine (Phila Pa 1976). 2000;25:389–94.
9. Akdemir G. Thoracic and lumbar intraforaminal ligaments. J Neurosurg Spine. 2010;13:351–5.
10. Jinkins JR, Whittemore AR, Bradley WG. The anatomic basis of vertebrogenic pain and the autonomic syndrome associated with lumbar disk extrusion. Am J Roentgenol. 1989;152:1277–89.
11. Lee JH, An JH, Lee SH. Comparison of the effectiveness of interlaminar and bilateral transforaminal epidural steroid injections in treatment of patients with lumbosacral disc herniation and spinal stenosis. Clin J Pain. 2009;25:206–10.
12. Sivaganesan A, Chotai S, Parker SL, Asher AL, McGirt MJ, Devin CJ. Predictors of the efficacy of epidural steroid injections for structural lumbar degenerative pathology. Spine J. 2016;16:928–34.
13. Lee JH, Lee SH. Clinical effectiveness of percutaneous adhesiolysis and predictive factors of treatment efficacy in patients with lumbosacral spinal stenosis. Pain Med. 2013;14:1497–504.
14. Park Y, Lee WY, Ahn JK, Nam HS, Lee KH. Percutaneous adhesiolysis versus transforaminal epidural steroid injection for the treatment of chronic radicular pain caused by lumbar foraminal spinal stenosis: a retrospective comparative study. Ann Rehabil Med. 2015;39:941–9.
15. Park CH, Lee SH. Effectiveness of percutaneous transforaminal adhesiolysis in patients with lumbar neuroforaminal spinal stenosis. Pain Physician. 2013;16:E37–43.

16. Kamihara M, Nakano S, Fukunaga T, Ikeda K, Tsunetoh T, Tanada D, et al. Spinal cord stimulation for treatment of leg pain associated with lumbar spinal stenosis. Neuromodulation. 2014;17:340–4. discussion 345
17. Costantini A, Buchser E, Van Buyten JP. Spinal cord stimulation for the treatment of chronic pain in patients with lumbar spinal stenosis. Neuromodulation. 2010;13:275–9. discussion 279–80
18. Soliman HM. Irrigation endoscopic decompressive laminotomy. A new endoscopic approach for spinal stenosis decompression. Spine J. 2015;15:2282–9.
19. Kim EH, Kim HT. En bloc partial laminectomy and posterior lumbar interbody fusion in foraminal spinal stenosis. Asian Spine J. 2009;3:66–72.
20. Haufe SM, Mork AR. Effects of unilateral endoscopic facetectomy on spinal stability. J Spinal Disord Tech. 2007;20:146–8.
21. Evins AI, Banu MA, Njoku I Jr, Elowitz EH, Härtl R, Bernado A, et al. Endoscopic lumbar foraminotomy. J Clin Neurosci. 2015;22:730–4.
22. Zaina F, Tomkins-Lane C, Carragee E, Negrini S. Surgical versus non-surgical treatment for lumbar spinal stenosis. Cochrane Database Syst Rev. 2016;2016:CD010264.
23. Yuan SG, Wen YL, Zhang P, Li YK. Ligament, nerve, and blood vessel anatomy of the lateral zone of the lumbar intervertebral foramina. Int Orthop. 2015;39:2135–41.
24. Park HK, Rudrappa S, Dujovny M, Diaz FG. Intervertebral foraminal ligaments of the lumbar spine: anatomy and biomechanics. Childs Nerv Syst. 2001;17:275–82.
25. Transfeldt EE, Robertson D, Bradford DS. Ligaments of the lumbosacral spine and their role in possible extraforaminal spinal nerve entrapment and tethering. J Spinal Disord. 1993;6:507–12.
26. Lee S, Lee JW, Yeom JS, Kim KJ, Kim HJ, Chung SK, et al. A practical MRI grading system for lumbar foraminal stenosis. Am J Roentgenol. 2010;194:1095–8.
27. Farrar JT, Young JP Jr, LaMoreaux L, Werth JL, Poole RM. Clinical importance of changes in chronic pain intensity measured on an 11-point numerical pain rating scale. Pain. 2001;94:149–58.
28. Jeon CH, Kim DJ, Kim SK, Kim DJ, Lee HM, Park HJ. Validation in the cross-cultural adaptation of the Korean version of the Oswestry disability index. J Korean Med Sci. 2006;21:1092–7.
29. Moon J, Kim YC, Park SY, Lee SC, Choi SP, Nahm FS, et al. Psychometric characteristics of the Korean version of the Roland-Morris disability questionnaire. J Korean Med Sci. 2011;26:1364–70.
30. Dworkin RH, Turk DC, Farrar JT, Haythornthwaite JA, Jensen MP, Katz NP, et al. Core outcome measures for chronic pain clinical trials: IMMPACT recommendations. Pain. 2005;113:9–19.
31. Choi SS, Lee JH, Kim D, Kim HK, Lee S, Song KJ, et al. Effectiveness and factors associated with epidural decompression and adhesiolysis using a balloon-inflatable catheter in chronic lumbar spinal stenosis: 1-year follow-up. Pain Med. 2016;17:476–87.
32. Chiarotto A, Maxwell LJ, Terwee CB, Wells GA, Tugwell P, Ostelo RW. Roland-Morris disability questionnaire and Oswestry disability index: which has better measurement properties for measuring physical functioning in nonspecific low back pain? Systematic review and meta-analysis. Phys Ther. 2016;96:1620–37.
33. Fairbank JC, Pynsent PB. The Oswestry disability index. Spine (Phila Pa 1976). 2000;25:2940–52. discussion 52
34. Lee SC, Kim WJ, Lee CS, Moon JY. Effectiveness of percutaneous lumbar extraforaminotomy in patients with lumbar foraminal spinal stenosis: a prospective, single-armed, observational pilot study. Pain Med. 2017;18:1975–86.
35. Roland M, Fairbank J. The Roland-Morris disability questionnaire and the Oswestry disability questionnaire. Spine (Phila Pa 1976). 2000;25:3115–24.

Motorized Percutaneous Foraminoplasty

12

Sung-Eun Sim and Yongjae Yoo

12.1 Introduction

Lumbar foraminal neuropathy is a pathological condition associated with a narrowed vertebral foramen that affects its neurovascular contents and causes radicular symptoms. Minimally invasive techniques with various devices are utilized to achieve effective and safe decompression of the lumbar spinal foramen. These techniques, such as percutaneous foraminoplasty with a paraspinal approach, facilitate direct access to foraminal lesions with the least manipulation of the facet joint and less postoperative pain than surgical decompression. Percutaneous foraminoplasty can be performed under local anesthesia, allowing direct feedback from the patient to avoid nerve damage during the procedure.

S.-E. Sim (✉)
Department of Anesthesiology and Pain Medicine, Seoul St. Mary's Hospital, Seoul, Republic of Korea

Y. Yoo
Department of Anesthesiology and Pain Medicine, Seoul National University Hospital, Seoul, Republic of Korea

S.-H. Lee (ed.), *Minimally Invasive Spine Interventions*,
https://doi.org/10.1007/978-981-16-9547-6_12

12.2 Background

Lumbar foraminal spinal stenosis (LFSS) is a common cause of lumbar radiculopathy, with a 10% incidence rate in the global population [1]. LFSS is defined as the narrowing of the vertebral foramen through which a nerve root passes associated with a herniated IVD [2–4], osteoarthritic changes in the facet joints, or a hypertrophied ligamentum flavum, which can provoke neurogenic claudication [5–7]. LFSS-related pain is thought to arise from the DRG that is impinged within the foramen, given the high concentration of substance P in the DRG [8] and its sensitivity to external pressure [9, 10].

LFSS-related pain can initially be managed with conservative treatment, including oral medications, ESIs, and physical therapy. However, patients who do not respond to those therapies are usually advised to undergo surgery as the next step. Conventional surgical methods for LFSS may be categorized into total or partial facetectomy, with or without fusion and facet-preserving foraminoplasty [11]. Of these techniques, facetectomy offers sufficient decompression around the nerve root; however, it often leads to segmental instability [6, 12, 13]. Moreover, this surgical approach requires general anesthesia and, occasionally, a long hospital stay and slow recovery; it also poses the risk of procedure-related complications [14, 15]. On the other hand, compared with conventional surgery, minimally invasive techniques, such as percutaneous foraminoplasty with a paraspinal approach, facilitate direct access to foraminal lesions with the least manipulation of the facet joint and less postoperative pain [16]. Percutaneous foraminoplasty can be performed under local anesthesia, allowing the patient to report neurological symptoms. This feedback minimizes the risk of nerve damage during the procedure [17].

12.3 Motorized Percutaneous Foraminoplasty

Foraminoplasty is the process of widening the foramen by undercutting the ventral part of the SAP and ablating the foraminal ligament using bone trephines or an endoscopic drill [18]. Although classified as a minimally invasive technique, percutaneous endoscopic foraminoplasty is a time-consuming procedure that requires a working channel for the rigid endoscope and expensive equipment and involves a steep learning curve [19]. In the mid-2000s, Schubert and Hoogland introduced percutaneous lumbar foraminoplasty (PLF) [20], a process in which transforaminal percutaneous reamers with a guidewire are used to drill to the tip of the SAP. During PLF, a trephine and a bone reamer allow rapid resection of the hypertrophied SAP or osteophyte under fluoroscopic guidance [21]. This method may be more convenient and time-saving than the endoscopic procedure; however, it entails safety issues, such as the risk of injury to the exiting and traversing nerve root, related to mechanical or thermal irritation during the procedure [22].

This potential for complications inspired Dr. Sim (author) to invent the Claudicare device, a specially designed motorized percutaneous foraminoplasty (MPF) instrument with a portable battery. The tool has a tip with a blunt end and a shield to protect the nerve root during the procedure. As the maximum outer diameter of the device is only 3.5 mm, MPF might be relatively non-traumatic and efficient. A previous study showed that MPF might be an optimal and safe option for managing intractable LFSS-related pain on an outpatient basis [23]. The NRS pain score and duration of walking without radicular pain were improved significantly from baseline at the three-month follow-up, and no serious adverse events occurred.

12.4 Indications for Percutaneous Foraminoplasty

1. Patients with radiculopathy and neurogenic claudication secondary to MRI-confirmed LFSS.
2. Predominant radicular or referred leg pain rather than LBP.
3. Persistent pain after receiving at least 3 months of conservative treatment, including oral medication, physical therapy, and ESIs.
4. Incomplete or short-term pain relief (<1 month) after a previous transforaminal ESI.

12.5 Contraindications

12.5.1 Absolute

1. Back pain in a setting suspicious for a severe underlying cause, such as cauda equina syndrome, cancer, fracture, and infection.
2. Allergies to local anesthetics or contrast dyes.
3. Pregnancy.
4. Coagulation disorder.
5. Local infection at the puncture site.

12.5.2 Relative

1. A large contained or sequestered disc herniation or severe central canal stenosis on lumbar MRI scans.
2. Segmental instability at the level of the symptomatic disc.

12.6 Complications

1. Pain at the incision site.

2. Infection at the incision site.
3. Hematoma.
4. Transient motor weakness or sensory change in the lower legs.

12.7 Preoperative Preparation

1. History and physical examination.
2. Imaging diagnosis: MRI or CT.
3. Other studies and issues.
   - Nerve conduction study and electromyography.
   - Complete blood count, coagulation panel, and urinalysis.
   - Antiplatelet agents and anticoagulants should be discontinued before and after the procedure according to recent consensus guidelines [24].

12.8 Operating Room Supplies

12.8.1 Instruments (Fig. 12.1)

1. Guidewire.
2. Dilator.
3. Working cannula.
4. Drill.
5. Portable, disposable battery.

12.8.2 Solutions

1. Lidocaine for skin infiltration.

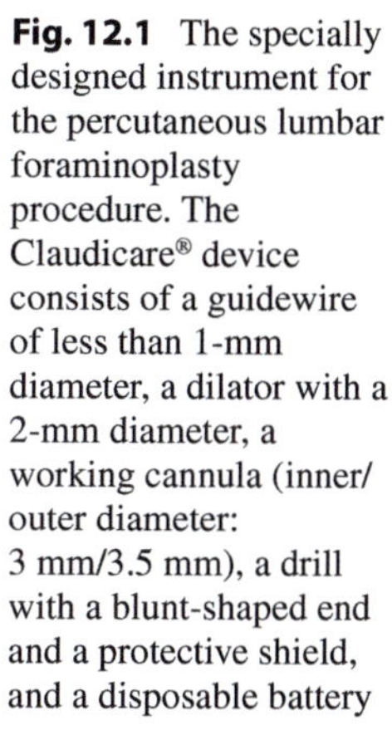

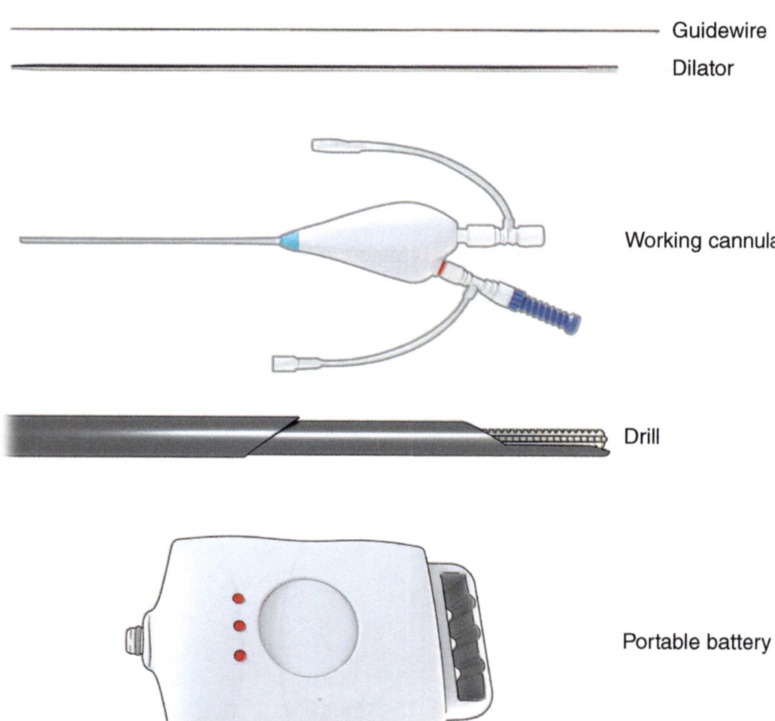

Fig. 12.1 The specially designed instrument for the percutaneous lumbar foraminoplasty procedure. The Claudicare® device consists of a guidewire of less than 1-mm diameter, a dilator with a 2-mm diameter, a working cannula (inner/outer diameter: 3 mm/3.5 mm), a drill with a blunt-shaped end and a protective shield, and a disposable battery

2. 0.125% bupivacaine or 0.2% ropivacaine
3. Contrast agent.
4. Optional: hyaluronidase and corticosteroids.

12.9 Procedure

- Step 1. The patient's written informed consent is obtained.
- Step 2. A pre-procedural prophylactic antibiotic injection should be considered (e.g., cefazolin 1 g IV).
- Step 3. The patient is placed in the prone position with a pillow under the lower abdomen to reduce lumbar lordosis.
- Step 4. Electrocardiography, heart rate, noninvasive blood pressure, and peripheral oxygen saturation are monitored during the procedure, and the patient is conscious throughout to report any changes in symptoms.
- Step 5. Sterile skin preparation and draping are performed.
- Step 6. C-arm fluoroscopy is used in the AP, oblique, and lateral planes to confirm the target disc, align the endplates of the vertebral bodies, and direct instrument placement on the disc surface.
- Step 7. Lidocaine (5–10 mL) is injected at the skin entry point approximately 8–10 cm off the midline and infiltrated throughout the needle trajectory, and then the skin is incised.
- Step 8. A guidewire is inserted into Kambin's triangle using a 45-degree ipsilateral oblique view (Fig. 12.2).
- Step 9. The guidewire is advanced until its tip is located at the SAP using the lateral fluoroscopic view (Fig. 12.3).
- Step 10. After touching the SAP with the guidewire, an AP image is obtained to confirm that the guidewire tip is located at the medial border of the SAP (Fig. 12.4).

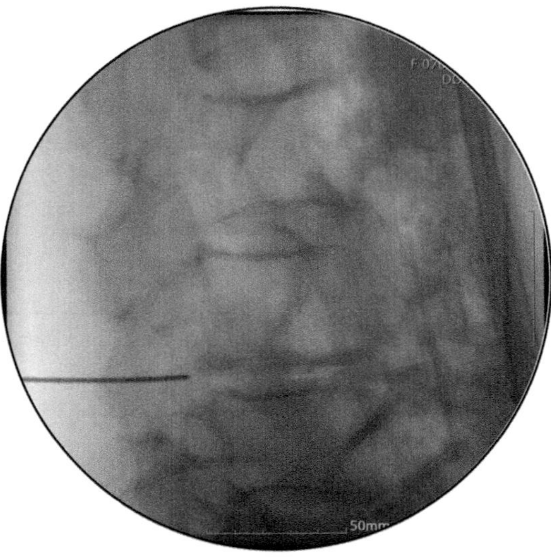

Fig. 12.3 Step 9. The lateral view of the tip

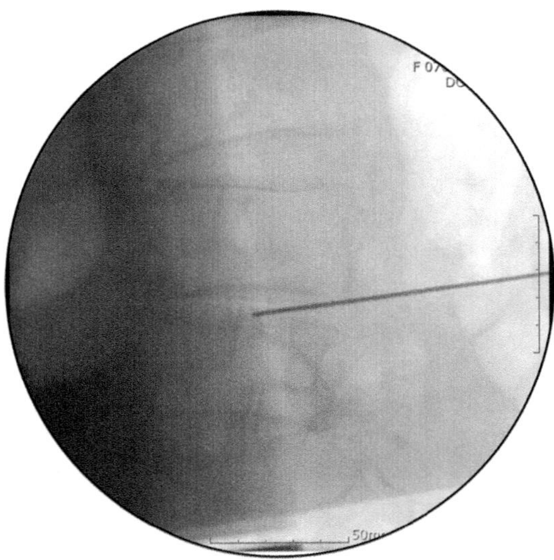

Fig. 12.2 Step 8. The guidewire tip is placed on Kambin's triangle

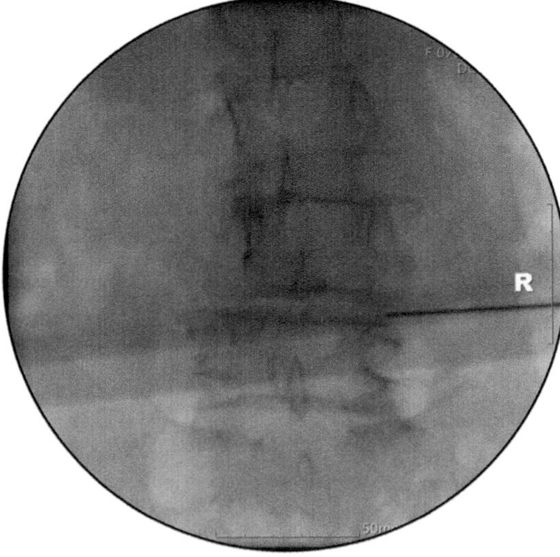

Fig. 12.4 Step 10. The guidewire tip is located at the medial border of the SAP

- Step 11. The guidewire is advanced approximately 0.5 cm anteriorly into the target epidural foramen in the lateral fluoroscopic view (Fig. 12.5).
- Step 12. A 2-mm-diameter dilator is advanced over the guidewire toward the target foramen until it touches the anterior border of the SAP (Fig. 12.6).
- Step 13. The guidewire is removed, and a working cannula with an outer diameter of 3.5 mm is inserted through the dilator and advanced to the anterior border of the hypertrophied SAP (Fig. 12.7a, b).
- Step 14. A drill with a shield on the tip is inserted through the working cannula and con-

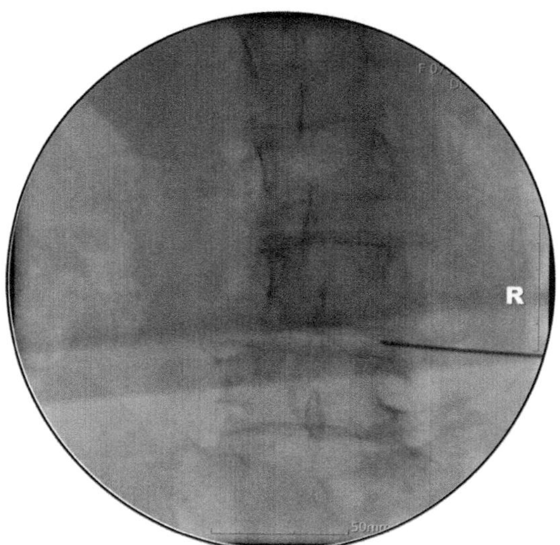

Fig. 12.5 Step 11. Gentle advancing guidewire tip

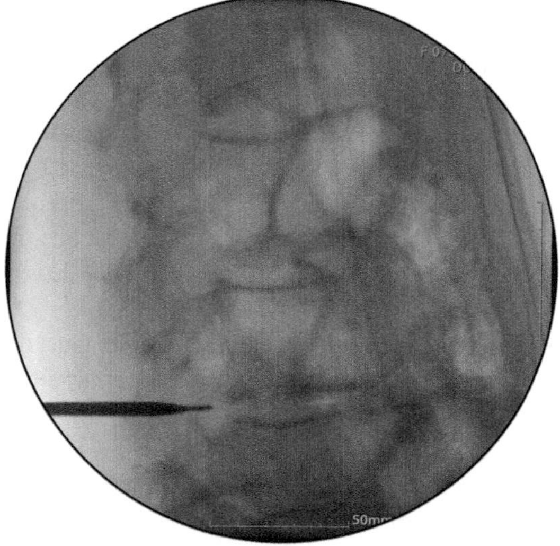

Fig. 12.6 Step 12. Insertion of a dilator

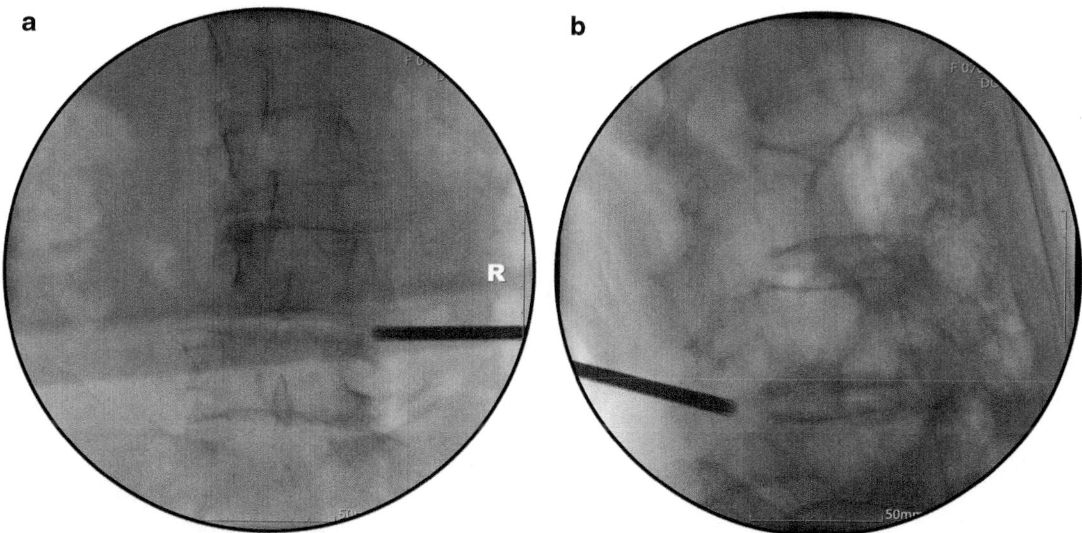

Fig. 12.7 Step 13. Placement of working cannula. Anterioposterior view (**a**), lateral view (**b**)

nected to a specially designed disposable battery.

- Step 15. After ensuring that the leg has no pain or motor defect, the hypertrophied SAP capsule is partially removed from the lateral to the medial direction in the AP fluoroscopic view using the drill at speeds ranging from 12,500 rpm (low-power mode) to 17,500 rpm (high-power mode) (Fig. 12.8a, b) while obtaining lateral fluoroscopy images to confirm the drill tip position.
- Step 16. After drilling back and forth approximately 3–5 times, a slight reduction in resistance to the drill tip should become apparent, with thinning of the anterior capsule of the SAP.
- Step 17. This process is repeated approximately 3–4 times until the drill tip reaches the medial border of the pedicle in the AP fluoroscopic view.
- Step 18. The drill tip shield should face the nerve root throughout the procedure to protect against nerve damage (Fig. 12.9).
- Step 19. As the hypertrophied SAP capsule and part of the thickened transforaminal ligament in the target foramen are drilled, the ground fragments of the capsule are removed through the working channel (Fig. 12.10).
- Step 20. Mild bleeding drains through the working channel due to the pressure gradient and usually stops spontaneously.
- Step 21. If needed, local anesthetics with or without hyaluronidase and steroids are administered directly to the pathological sites (Fig. 12.11).
- Step 22. If necessary, a catheter is advanced through the working channel to the targeted nerve to allow the injection of local anesthetics with or without steroid.

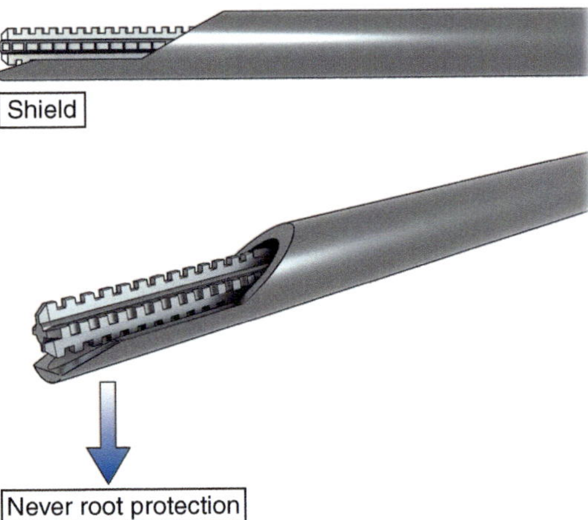

Fig. 12.9 Step 18. Positioning of the shield of drill

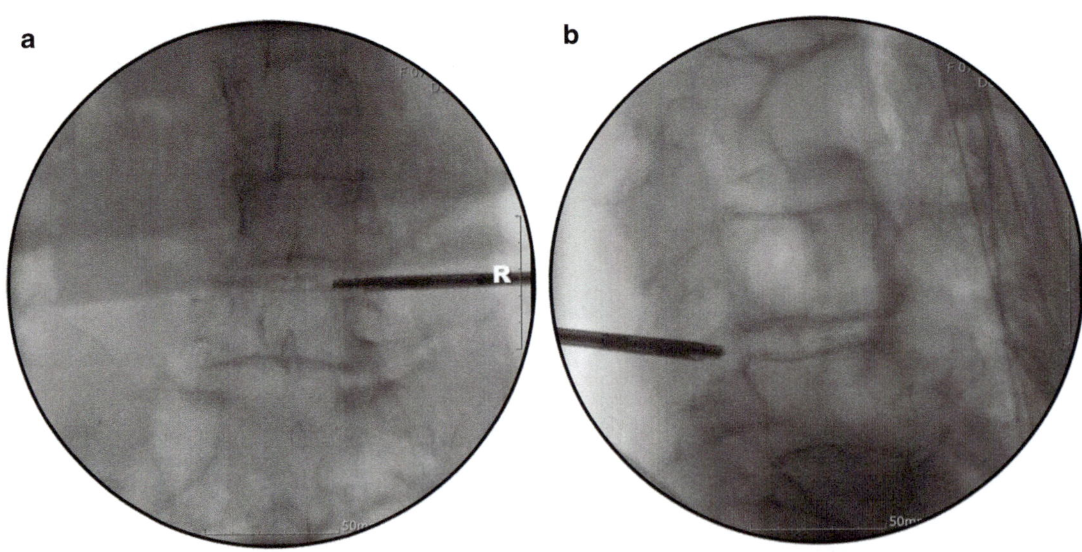

Fig. 12.8 Step 15. Drilling carefully. Anterioposterior view (**a**), lateral view (**b**)

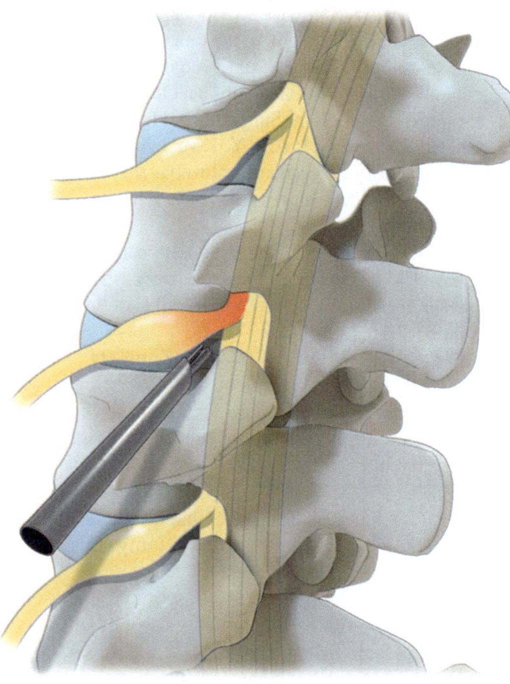

Fig. 12.10 Step 19. The mimetic illustration of the drilling procedure

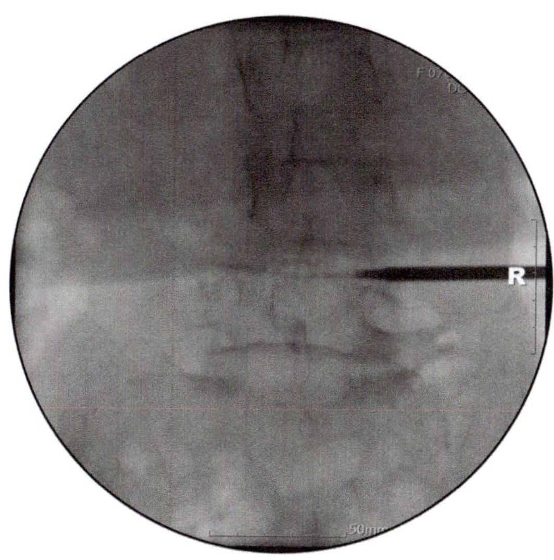

Fig. 12.11 Step 21. Injections

- Step 23. In cases of continuous bleeding, a Jackson-Pratt drain can be placed and retained for several hours until hemostasis occurs.
- Step 24. The working channel is removed.
- Step 25. The skin is sutured, and a sterile dressing is applied.

12.10 Postprocedural Management

1. A postoperative neurologic examination should be performed; if a new neurologic deficit is detected, MRI and a neurology consultation should be considered.
2. The patient is instructed not to bathe until the suture is removed.
3. Appropriate analgesics are prescribed.
4. Prophylactic antibiotics are administered for 3 days.

12.11 Conclusions

MPF using the Claudicare device is an outpatient procedure that could reduce the symptoms of lumbar foraminal stenosis; the expected benefits include diminished pain and improved motor function, including increased duration of walking without radicular pain. The rates of procedure-related discomfort and adverse events were reportedly trivial.

References

1. Ishimoto Y, Yoshimura N, Muraki S, Yamada H, Nagata K, Hashizume H, et al. Prevalence of symptomatic lumbar spinal stenosis and its association with physical performance in a population-based cohort in Japan: the Wakayama Spine Study. Osteoarthr Cartil. 2012;20:1103–8.
2. Kunogi J, Hasue M. Diagnosis and operative treatment of intraforaminal and extraforaminal nerve root compression. Spine (Phila Pa 1976). 1991;16:1312–20.
3. Lee SY, Kim TH, Oh JK, Lee SJ, Park MS. Lumbar stenosis: a recent update by review of literature. Asian Spine J. 2015;9:818–28.
4. Porter RW, Hibbert C, Evans C. The natural history of root entrapment syndrome. Spine (Phila Pa 1976). 1984;9:418–21.
5. Hasegawa T, An HS, Haughton VM, Nowicki BH. Lumbar foraminal stenosis: critical heights of

the intervertebral discs and foramina. A cryomicrotome study in cadavera. J Bone Joint Surg Am. 1995;77:32–8.
6. Jenis LG, An HS. Spine update. Lumbar foraminal stenosis. Spine (Phila Pa 1976). 2000;25:389–94.
7. Splendiani A, Ferrari F, Barile A, Masciocchi C, Gallucci M. Occult neural foraminal stenosis caused by association between disc degeneration and facet joint osteoarthritis: demonstration with dedicated upright MRI system. Radiol Med. 2014;119:164–74.
8. Kobayashi S, Kokubo Y, Uchida K, Yayama T, Takeno K, Negoro K, et al. Effect of lumbar nerve root compression on primary sensory neurons and their central branches: changes in the nociceptive neuropeptides substance P and somatostatin. Spine (Phila Pa 1976). 2005;30:276–82.
9. Vanderlinden RG. Subarticular entrapment of the dorsal root ganglion as a cause of sciatic pain. Spine (Phila Pa 1976). 1984;9:19–22.
10. Weinstein J. Report of the 1985 ISSLS traveling fellowship. Mechanisms of spinal pain. The dorsal root ganglion and its role as a mediator of low-back pain. Spine (Phila Pa 1976). 1986;11:999–1001.
11. Ahn Y, Oh HK, Kim H, Lee SH, Lee HN. Percutaneous endoscopic lumbar foraminotomy: an advanced surgical technique and clinical outcomes. Neurosurgery. 2014;75:124–33. discussion 132–3
12. Abumi K, Panjabi MM, Kramer KM, Duranceau J, Oxland T, Crisco JJ. Biomechanical evaluation of lumbar spinal stability after graded facetectomies. Spine (Phila Pa 1976). 1990;15:1142–7.
13. Epstein NE. Foraminal and far lateral lumbar disc herniations: surgical alternatives and outcome measures. Spinal Cord. 2002;40:491–500.
14. Polikandriotis JA, Hudak EM, Perry MW. Minimally invasive surgery through endoscopic laminotomy and foraminotomy for the treatment of lumbar spinal stenosis. J Orthop. 2013;10:13–6.
15. Schoenfeld AJ, Ochoa LM, Bader JO, Belmont PJ Jr. Risk factors for immediate postoperative complications and mortality following spine surgery: a study of 3475 patients from the National Surgical Quality Improvement Program. J Bone Joint Surg Am. 2011;93:1577–82.
16. Chang SB, Lee SH, Ahn Y, Kim JM. Risk factor for unsatisfactory outcome after lumbar foraminal and far lateral microdecompression. Spine (Phila Pa 1976). 2006;31:1163–7.
17. Chun EH, Park HS. A modified approach of percutaneous endoscopic lumbar discectomy (PELD) for far lateral disc herniation at L5-S1 with foot drop. Korean J Pain. 2016;29:57–61.
18. Choi G, Lee SH, Lokhande P, Kong BJ, Shim JS, Jung B, et al. Percutaneous endoscopic approach for highly migrated intracanal disc herniations by foraminoplastic technique using rigid working channel endoscope. Spine (Phila Pa 1976). 2008;33:E508–15.
19. Hsu HT, Chang SJ, Yang SS, Chai CL. Learning curve of full-endoscopic lumbar discectomy. Eur Spine J. 2013;22:727–33.
20. Schubert M, Hoogland T. Endoscopic transforaminal nucleotomy with foraminoplasty for lumbar disk herniation. Oper Orthop Traumatol. 2005;17:641–61.
21. Li ZZ, Hou SX, Shang WL, Song KR, Zhao HL. Modified percutaneous lumbar foraminoplasty and percutaneous endoscopic lumbar discectomy: instrument design, technique notes, and 5 years follow-up. Pain Physician. 2017;20:E85–98.
22. Sencer A, Yorukoglu AG, Akcakaya MO, Aras Y, Aydoseli A, Boyali O, et al. Fully endoscopic interlaminar and transforaminal lumbar discectomy: short-term clinical results of 163 surgically treated patients. World Neurosurg. 2014;82:884–90.
23. Yoo Y, Moon JY, Yoon S, Kwon SM, Sim SE. Clinical outcome of percutaneous lumbar foraminoplasty using a safety-improved device in patients with lumbar foraminal spinal stenosis. Medicine (Baltimore). 2019;98:e15169.

13 Conclusion

Sang-Heon Lee

The evolution of fluoroscopically guided procedures to help diagnose and manage pain due to the spine began in the late 1970s and gradually became the standard of practice in the late 1990s. Likewise, the evolution of endoscopic disc surgery started in the late 1980s and the early 1990s. However, its widespread acceptance took longer, likely paralleling the more gradual improvement in endoscopic optics [1].

All minimally invasive procedures aim to achieve comparative outcomes at lower morbidity and cost—arguably reached for the endoscopic approach to herniated discs nerve root compression with radicular pain caused by herniated disc herniation [1].

The editors asked physicians to detail their indications, risks, and techniques for minimally invasive procedures. If their topic included specific devices, the editors specifically chose published experts who were either inventors or participated in early device development. The editors concede that the published studies and meta-analyses on many minimally invasive procedures are biased. An author may pick the study that validates one's own bias—including this author.

Few of the procedures covered are slam-dunks. As a general rule, even when treating conditions generally thought to have robust outcomes, such as radicular pain due to a herniated disc, the chance of the patient never complaining about ongoing or recurrent pain is probably at or below 50% than to the often quoted 80% to 90% [2].

Furthermore, most have a significant risk of adverse outcomes if one ignores authors' contraindications or technical safeguards. When assessing patient risk versus benefits, an interventionalist must include one own training to handle complications, available backup by specialists, and the surgical setting. For example, a non-surgeon interventionalist hesitated before deciding to use Dr. Lee's epidural approach to extruded disc fragments with subsequent ablation because he mostly worked without immediately available surgical backup outside a hospital setting.

The book provides the reader with an introduction and technical reference to essential needle and important emerging cannula and endoscopic surgical procedures. All discussed techniques have a steep learning curve. Finally, unless an expert in closely related techniques, one must not perform the described operations based solely on the written descriptions.

S.-H. Lee (✉)
Department of Spine and Pain Center, Korea
University Anam Hospital, Seoul, Republic of Korea

S.-H. Lee (ed.), *Minimally Invasive Spine Interventions*,
https://doi.org/10.1007/978-981-16-9547-6_13

References

1. Birkenmaier C, Komp M, Leu HF, Wegener B, Ruetten S. The current state of endoscopic disc surgery: review of controlled studies comparing full-endoscopic procedures for disc herniations to standard procedures. Pain Physician. 2013;16(4):335–44.
2. Bokov A, Isrelov A, Skorodumov A, Aleynik A, Simonov A, Mlyavykh S. An analysis of reasons for failed back surgery syndrome and partial results after different types of surgical lumbar nerve root decompression. Pain Physician. 2011;14:545–57.

Batch number: 10371059

Printed by Printforce, the Netherlands